# *Curren*

# Surgery

1997 Edition

## The University of California, Irvine Manual of Surgery

### Samuel Eric Wilson, M.D.
Professor and Chairman
Department of Surgery
College of Medicine
University of California, Irvine

**James G. Jakowatz, M.D.**
**John A. Butler, M.D.**
**Charles F. Chandler, M.D.**
**Bruce M. Achauer, M.D.**
**I. James Sarfeh, M.D.**
**Paul D. Chan, M.D.**
**David A. Chamberlin, M.D.**
**J. Craig Collins, M.D.**
**C. Garo Gholdoian, M.D.**
**Ian L. Gordon, M.D., Ph.D.**
**Joshua Helman, M.D.**
**Fernando Kafie, M.D.**
**Harry Skinner, M.D.**
**Russell A. Williams, M.D.**

Copyright © 1997 CCS Publishing. All rights reserved.

This book, or any parts thereof, may not be reproduced, photocopied, or stored in an information retrieval network without the permission of the publisher. The reader is advised to consult the drug package insert and other references before using any therapeutic agent. The publisher disclaims any liability, loss, injury, or damage incurred as a consequence, directly or indirectly, of the use and application of any of the contents of this text. Current Clinical Strategies is a trademark of CCS Publishing.

**Current Clinical Strategies Publishing, Inc.**
27071 Cabot Road, Suite 126
Laguna Hills, California 92653
**Phone:** 800-331-8227 or 714-348-8404
**Fax:** 800-965-9420 or 714-348-8405
**Internet:** http://www.CCSPublishing.com
**E-mail:** CCSPublishing@msn.com

Printed in USA

ISBN 1-881528-28-6

# Contents

**Surgical Documentation** .................................................. 5
  Surgical History and Physical Examination ........................ 5
  Preoperative Preparation of the Surgical Patient ................. 6
  Admitting and Preoperative Orders ................................ 7
  Preoperative Note ................................................ 8
  Brief Operative Note ............................................. 8
  Operative Report ................................................. 9
  Post-Operative Note .............................................. 9
  Post-Operative Orders ............................................ 9
  Post-Operative Management ....................................... 10
  Problem-Oriented Surgical Progress Note ......................... 10
  Discharge Summary ............................................... 11

**Clinical Care of the Surgical Patient** ................................. 12
  Blood Component Therapy ......................................... 12
  Fluids and Electrolytes ......................................... 13
  Evaluation of Postoperative Fever ............................... 14
  Sepsis .......................................................... 15
  Enteral Nutrition ............................................... 19
  Parenteral Nutrition ............................................ 19
  Central Venous Catheterization .................................. 21
  Pulmonary Artery Catheterization ................................ 22
  Normal Pulmonary Artery Catheter Values ......................... 23
  Venous Cutdown .................................................. 23
  Arterial Line Placement ......................................... 24
  Cricothyrotomy .................................................. 24

**Trauma** ............................................................... 27
  Management of the Trauma Patient ................................ 27
  Abdominal Trauma ................................................ 28
  Penetrating Abdominal Trauma .................................... 29
  Blunt Abdominal Trauma .......................................... 29
  Diagnostic Peritoneal Lavage .................................... 30
  Head Trauma ..................................................... 31
  Pneumothorax .................................................... 32
  Tension Pneumothorax ............................................ 33
  Flail Chest ..................................................... 34
  Massive Hemothorax .............................................. 35
  Cardiac Tamponade ............................................... 35
  Pericardiocentesis .............................................. 36
  Other Life-Threatening Trauma Emergencies ....................... 37
    Cardiac Contusions ......................................... 37
    Pulmonary Contusions ....................................... 37
    Traumatic Aortic Transection ............................... 37
    Pelvic Fracture ............................................ 37
    Extremity Fractures: ....................................... 37
    Traumatic Esophageal Injuries .............................. 37
  Burns ........................................................... 38

**Pulmonology** .......................................................... 41
  Airway Management and Intubation ................................ 41
  Ventilator Management ........................................... 42

Epistaxis ........................................... 44

## Disorders of the Alimentary Tract ............................ 49
Acute Abdomen ....................................... 49
Management of the Acute Abdomen ........................ 51
Appendicitis ......................................... 52
Appendectomy Surgical Technique ........................ 53
Abdominal Hernias .................................... 54
Evaluation of the Hernia Patient .......................... 55
Surgical Repair Techniques for Hernias .................... 55
Hernia Repair Technique ................................ 56
Hematemesis and Upper Gastrointestinal Bleeding ........... 58
Variceal Bleeding ..................................... 59
Peptic Ulcer Disease .................................. 61
Lower Gastrointestinal Bleeding .......................... 64
Anorectal Disorders ................................... 68
    Anal Fissures ..................................... 69
    Perianal Abscess .................................. 69
    Condylomata Acuminata ............................. 70
Fistula-in-Ano ........................................ 71
Colorectal Cancer .................................... 71
Mesenteric Ischemia and Infarction ....................... 74
Intestinal Obstruction .................................. 75
Acute Pancreatitis .................................... 76
Cholecystitis and Cholelithiasis .......................... 80
Management of the Cholecystectomy Patient ............... 81
Laparoscopic Cholecystectomy Procedure ................. 82
Open Cholecystectomy Procedure ........................ 82

## Breast Cancer ............................................. 85
Evaluation of Breast Masses ............................ 85
Excisional Breast Biopsy ............................... 87

## Urology .................................................. 88
Prostate Cancer ...................................... 88
Renal Colic .......................................... 90
Urologic Emergencies ................................. 92
    Acute Urinary Retention ............................. 92
    Testicular Torsion .................................. 94
    Priapism .......................................... 95

## Vascular and Orthopedic Surgery ............................ 97
Peripheral Arterial Disease ............................. 97
Deep Venous Thrombosis .............................. 100
Orthopedic Fractures and Dislocations ................... 103

## References ............................................... 106

## Index .................................................... 107

Surgical History and Physical Examination

# *Surgical Documentation*

## Surgical History and Physical Examination

**Identifying Data:** Patient's name, age, race, sex; referring physician; hospital identification number.

**Chief Compliant:** Reason given by patient for seeking surgical care; place patient's complaint in quotation marks.

**History of Present Illness (HPI):** Describe the course of the patient's illness, including when it began, character of the symptoms; pain onset (gradual or rapid), precise character of pain (constant, intermittent, cramping, stabbing, radiating); other factors associated with pain (defecation, urination, eating, strenuous activities); location where the symptoms began; aggravating or relieving factors. Vomiting (color, content, blood, coffee-ground emesis, frequency, associated pain). Change in bowel habits; bleeding, character of blood (clots, bright or dark red), trauma; recent weight loss or anorexia; other related diseases; past diagnostic testing.

**Past Medical History (PMH):** Past medical problems. Previous operations and indications; dates and types of procedures; serious injuries, hospitalizations; diabetes, hypertension, peptic ulcer disease, asthma, heart disease; hernia, gallstones.

**Medications:** Aspirin, anticoagulants, hypertensive and cardiac medications, diuretics, anticonvulsants.

**Allergies:** Penicillin, codeine, iodine, others.

**Family History:** Medical problems in relatives. Family history of colonic polyposis, carcinomas.

**Social History:** Alcohol, smoking, drug usage, occupation.

**Review of Systems (ROS):**

**General:** Weight gain or loss; loss of appetite, fever, fatigue, night sweats. Activity level.

**HEENT:** Headaches, seizures, sore throat, masses, dentures.

**Respiratory:** Cough, sputum, hemoptysis, dyspnea on exertion, ability to walk up flight of stairs.

**Cardiovascular:** Chest pain, orthopnea, claudication, extremity edema.

**Gastrointestinal:** Dysphagia, vomiting, abdominal pain, hematemesis, melena (black tarry stools), hematochezia (bright red blood per rectum), constipation, change in bowel habits; hernia, hemorrhoids, gallstones.

**Genitourinary:** Dysuria, hesitancy, hematuria, discharge; impotence, prostate problems.

**Gynecological:** Last menstrual period, gravida, para, abortions, length of regular cycle birth control.

**Skin:** Easy bruising, bleeding tendencies.

**Neurological:** Stroke, transient ischemic attacks, weakness.


### Surgical Physical Examination

**Vital Signs:** Temperature, respirations, heart rate, blood pressure, weight.
**Eyes:** Pupils equally round and react to light and accommodation (PERRLA); extraocular movements intact (EOMI).

**Neck:** Jugular venous distention (JVD), thyromegaly, masses, bruits; lymphadenopathy; trachea midline.
**Chest:** Equal expansion, dullness to percussion; rales, rhonchi, breath sounds.
**Heart:** Regular rate and rhythm (RRR), first and second heart sounds; murmurs (grade 1-6), pulses (graded 0-2+).
**Breast:** Skin retractions, tenderness, masses (mobile, fixed) nipple discharge, erythema, axillary or supraclavicular node enlargement.
**Abdomen:** Contour (flat, scaphoid, obese, distended); scars, bowel sounds, bruits, tenderness, masses, liver span; splenomegaly, guarding, rebound, percussion note (tympanic), pulsatile masses, costovertebral angle tenderness (CVAT), abdominal hernias.
**Genitourinary:** Inguinal hernias, testicles, varicoceles; urethral discharge.
**Extremities:** Edema (grade 1-4+); cyanosis, clubbing, pulses (radial, ulnar, femoral, popliteal, posterior tibial, dorsalis pedis; simultaneous palpation of radial and femoral pulses). Grading of pulses: 0 = absent; 1+ weak; 2+ normal; 3+ very strong.
**Rectal Exam:** Masses, tenderness hemorrhoids, guaiac test for occult blood; prostate masses; bimanual palpation.
**Neurological:** Mental status; gait, strength (graded 0-5); tendon reflexes, sensory testing.
**Laboratory Evaluation:** Electrolytes (sodium, potassium, bicarbonate, chloride, BUN, creatinine), blood glucose, liver function tests, PT/PTT, CBC with differential; X-rays, ECG (if older than 35 yrs or cardiovascular disease), urine analysis.
**Assessment (Impression):** Assign a number to each problem and discuss each problem separately. Begin with most important problem and rank in order.
**Plan:** Discuss surgical plans for each numbered problem, including preoperative testing, laboratory studies, medications, antibiotics, preoperative endoscopy.

# Preoperative Preparation of the Surgical Patient

1. Review patient's history and physical examination, and write a preoperative note assessing patient's overall condition and operative risk.
2. **Preoperative Laboratory Evaluation:** Electrolytes, BUN, creatinine, PT/PTT, CBC, platelet count, UA, ABG, pulmonary function test. Chest X-ray (if patient has not had a normal chest x-ray in past 6 months or if >35 yrs old), EKG, (if older then 35 yrs old or if cardiovascular disease). Type and screen for an appropriate number of units of blood.
3. **Skin Preparation:** Patient to shower, and scrub the operative site with germicidal soap (Hibiclens) on the night before surgery. On the day of surgery, hair should be removed with an electric clipper or shaved just prior to operation.
4. **Prophylactic Antibiotics or Endocarditis Prophylaxis If Indicated.**
5. **Preoperative Incentive Spirometry** on the evening prior to surgery may be indicated for patients with pulmonary disease.
6. **Thromboembolic** prophylaxis should be provided for high-risk patients.
7. **Diet:** NPO after midnight.
8. **IV and Monitoring Lines:** At least one 18-gauge IV for initiation of anesthesia. Arterial catheter and pulmonary artery catheters (Swan-Ganz) if indicated. Patient to void on call to operating room.

9. **Medications**
   Preoperative sedation as ordered by anesthesiologist. Maintenance medications to be given the morning of surgery with a sip of water. Diabetics should receive one half of their usual AM insulin dose, and a insulin drip should be initiated with hourly glucose monitoring.
10. **Bowel Preparation**
    Bowel preparation is required for upper or lower GI tract procedures.
    **Antibiotic Preparation for Colonic Surgery**
    **Mechanical Prep:** Day 1: Clear liquid diet, laxative (milk of magnesia 30 cc or magnesium citrate 250 cc), tap water or Fleet enemas until clear. Day 2: Clear liquid diet, NPO, laxative. Day 3: Operation.
    **Whole Gut Lavage:** Polyethylene glycol electrolyte solution (GoLytely). Day 1: 2 liters PO or per nasogastric tube over 5 hours. Consider adding metoclopramide (Reglan) 10 mg PO prn nausea; clear liquid diet. Day 2: Operation.
    **Oral Antibiotic Prep:** One day prior to surgery, after mechanical or whole gut lavage, give neomycin 1 gm and erythromycin 1 gm PO at 1 p.m., 2 p.m., 11 p.m. May substitute metronidazole 500 mg PO for erythromycin.
11. **Preoperative IV Antibiotics:** Initiated immediately preoperatively; consider additional dose during operation and 1 dose of antibiotic postoperatively to 24 hours post-op. Cefotetan (every 12 hours) for bowel flora, or first generation cephalosporin (Cefazolin) for clean procedures.
12. **Anticoagulants:** Discontinue Coumadin; stop IV heparin 6 hours prior to surgery.
13. **Consider Stress Dose Steroids:** Hydrocortisone 100 mg at midnight and at induction if history of steroid medication.

# Admitting and Preoperative Orders

**Admit to:** Ward, ICU, or preoperative room.
**Diagnosis:** Intended operation and indication.
**Condition:**
**Vital Signs:** Frequency of vital signs; input and output recording; neurological or vascular checks. Notify physician if blood pressure <90/60, >160/110; pulse >110; pulse <60; temperature >101.5; urine output <35 cc/h for >2 hours; respiratory rate >30.
**Activity:** Bed rest or ambulation; bathroom privileges.
**Allergies:**
**Diet:** NPO
**IV Orders:** D5 1/2 NS at 100 cc/hour.
**Oxygen:** 6 L/min by nasal canula.
**Drains:** Foley catheter to closed drainage. Nasogastric tube with instructions for type of suction. Other drains, tubes, dressing changes. Orders for irrigation of tubes as appropriate.
**Medications:** Antibiotics to be initiated immediately preoperatively; consider additional dose during operation and 1 dose of antibiotic postoperatively to 24 hours post-op. Cefotetan (every 12 hours) for bowel flora, or first generation cephalosporin (Cefazolin) for clean procedures.
**Labs and Special X-Rays:** Electrolytes, BUN, creatinine, PT/PTT, CBC, platelet count, UA, ABG, pulmonary function test. Chest X-ray (if patient has not

had a normal chest x-ray in past 6 months or if >35 yrs old), EKG, (if older then 35 yrs old or if cardiovascular disease). Type and screen for an appropriate number of units of blood.

# Preoperative Note

**Preoperative Diagnosis:**
**Procedure Planned:**
**Type of Anesthesia Planned:**
**Laboratory Data:** Electrolytes, BUN, creatinine, CBC, PT/PTT, UA, EKG, Chest X-ray; type and screen for blood or cross match if indicated; liver function tests, ABG.
**Risk Factors:** Cardiovascular, pulmonary, hepatic, renal, coagulopathic, nutritional risk factors.
**American Surgical Association (ASA) grading (I-V) of surgical risk:** 1= normal; 2= mild systemic disease; 3= severe systemic disease; 4= disease with major threat to life; 5= not expected to survive.
**Consent:** Document explanation to patient of risk and benefits of procedure, and document patient's or guardian's informed consent and understanding of the procedure. Obtain signed consent form.
**Allergies:**
**Major Medical Problems:**
**Medications:**
**Special Requirements:** Signed blood transfusion consent form; documentation that patient with breast procedure has been given information brochure.

# Brief Operative Note

This note should be written in chart immediately after the surgical procedure.
**Date of the Procedure:**
**Preoperative Diagnosis:**
**Postoperative Diagnosis:**
**Procedure:**
**Operative Findings:**
**Names of Surgeon and Assistant:**
**Anesthesia:** General endotracheal, spinal, epidural, regional or local.
**Estimated Blood Loss (EBL):**
**Fluids and Blood Products Administered During Procedure:**
**Urine output:**
**Specimens:** Pathology specimens, cultures, blood samples.
**Intraoperative X-rays:**
**Drains:**

# Operative Report

This report should be dictated at the conclusion of surgical procedure.
**Identifying Data:** Name of patient, medical record number; name of dictating physician, date of dictation.
**Attending Surgeon and Service:**
**Date of Procedure:**
**Preoperative Diagnosis:**
**Postoperative Diagnosis:**
**Procedure Performed:**
**Names of Surgeon and Assistants:**
**Type of Anesthesia Used:**
**Estimated Blood Loss (EBL):**
**Fluid and Blood Products Administered During Operation:**
**Specimens:** Pathology, cultures, blood samples.
**Drains and Tubes Placed:**
**Complications:**
**Consultations Intraoperatively:**
**Indications for Surgery:** Brief history of patient and indications for surgery.
**Findings:**
**Description of Operation:** Position of patient; skin prep and draping; location and types of incisions; details of procedure from beginning to end including description of findings, both normal and abnormal, during surgery. Intraoperative studies or x-rays; hemostatic and closure techniques; dressings applied. Patient's condition and disposition. Needle and sponge counts as reported by operative nurse. Send copies of report to surgeons and referring physicians.

# Post-Operative Note

**Subjective:** Patient's mental status and subjective condition; adequacy of pain control.
**Objective:**
    **Vital Signs:** Temperature, blood pressure, pulse, respirations
    **Physical Exam:** Chest and lungs; inspection of wound and surgical dressings; condition of drains; characteristics and volume of output of drains.
    **Labs:** Hematocrit
**Assessment:** Make an assessment of the patient's overall condition and status of wound.
**Plan:** Describe post operative and discharge plans.

# Post-Operative Orders

1. **Transfer:** From recovery room to surgical ward when stable.
2. **Vital Signs:** q4h, I&O q4h x 24h.
3. **Activity:** Bed rest; ambulate in 6-8 hours if appropriate. Incentive spirometer q1h while awake.
4. **Diet:** NPO x 8h, then sips of water. Advance from clear liquids to regular diet as tolerated.

## 10 Post-Operative Management

5. **IV Fluids:** IV D5 LR or D5 1/2 NS at 125 cc/h (KCL, 20 mEq/L if indicated), Foley to gravity.
6. **Medications:**
   Cefazolin (Ancef) 1 gm IVPB q8h x 3 doses; if indicated for prophylaxis in clean cases **OR**
   Cefotetan 1 gm IV q12h x 2 doses for clean contaminated cases.
   Meperidine (Demerol) 50-75 mg IM q3-4h prn pain
   Hydroxyzine (Vistaril) 25-50 mg IM q3-4h prn pain **OR**
   Prochlorperazine (Compazine) 10 mg IM q4-6h prn nausea or suppository q 4h prn.
7. **Laboratory Evaluation:** CBC, SMA7, chest x-ray in AM if indicated.

# Post-Operative Management

I. **Post Op Day #1**
   A. Assess pain, lungs, cardiac status; flatulence, bowel movement. Examine for distension, tenderness, bowel sounds; wound drainage, bleeding from incision.
   B. Discontinue IV infusion when taking adequate PO fluids. Discontinue Foley catheter, and use in-and-out catheterization as needed for urinary retention as needed.
   C. Ambulate as tolerated; incentive spirometer, hematocrit and hemoglobin.
   D. Acetaminophen/codeine (Tylenol #3) 1-2 PO q4-6h prn pain.
   E. Colace 100 mg PO bid.
   F. Consider prophylaxis for deep vein thrombosis.

II. **Post Op Day #2**
   A. If passing gas or if bowel movement, advance to regular diet unless bowel resection.
   B. Laxatives: Dulcolax supp prn, or milk of magnesia, 30 cc PO prn.

III. **Post Op Day #3-7**
   A. Check pathology report.
   B. Consider removal of staples and placement of steri-strips.
   C. Consider discharge home on appropriate medications; follow up in 1-2 weeks for removal of staples or sutures.
   D. Write discharge orders (including prescriptions) early in AM; arrange for home health care if indicated. Dictate discharge summary and send copy to surgeon and referring physician.

# Problem-Oriented Surgical Progress Note

**Problem List:** Post-operative day number, antibiotic day number, hyperalimentation day number if applicable. List each surgical problem separately (e.g. status-post appendectomy, hypokalemia).
**Subjective:** Describe how the patient feels in the patient's own words; and give observations about the patient.
**Objective:** Vital signs; physical exam for each system; thorough examination and description of wound. Condition of dressings; purulent drainage, granulation

tissue, erythema; condition of sutures, dehiscence. Amount and color of drainage, laboratory data.
**Assessment:** Evaluate each numbered problem separately.
**Plan:** For each numbered problem, discuss any additional orders or surgical plans. Discuss changes in drug regimen or plans for discharge or transfer. Acknowledge conclusions of consultants.

# Discharge Summary

**Patient's Name:**
**Chart Number:**
**Date of Admission:**
**Date of Discharge:**
**Admitting Diagnosis:**
**Discharge Diagnosis:**
**Name of Attending or Ward Service:**
**Surgical Procedures, Diagnostic Tests, Invasive Procedures:**
**Brief History and Pertinent Physical Examination and Laboratory Data:** Describe the course of the disease up to the time the patient came to the hospital, and describe the physical exam and laboratory data on admission.
**Hospital Course:** Describe the course of the patient's illness while in the hospital, including evaluation, treatment, outcome of treatment, and medications given while in the hospital.
**Discharged Condition:** Describe improvement or deterioration in condition.
**Disposition:** Describe the situation to which the patient will be discharged (home, nursing home), and person who will provide care.
**Discharged Medications:** List medications and instructions (and write prescriptions).
**Discharged Instructions and Follow-up Care:** Date of return for follow-up care at clinic; diet, exercise instructions.
**Problem List:** List all active and past problems.
**Copies:** Send copies to attending physician, clinic, consultants and referring physician.

## 12 Radiographic Evaluation of Common Interventions

# *Clinical Care of the Surgical Patient*

James G. Jakowatz, M.D.

## Radiographic Evaluation of Common Interventions

I. **Central Intravenous Lines**
   A. **Central Venous Catheters** should be located above the right atrium in the superior vena cava, and not in a neck vein; the superior vena cava joins right atrium at level of right third costal cartilage. Rule out pneumothorax by checking chest x-ray and verifying that the lung markings extend completely to the rib cages on both sides (an upright, expiratory x-ray may be helpful). Examine for hydropericardium ("water bottle" sign, mediastinal widening). Do not attempt a second central line on the opposite side until chest x-ray shows no pneumothorax.
   B. **Pulmonary Artery Catheters** should be located centrally and posteriorly, and not more than 3-5 cm from midline. Do not attempt a second central line on the opposite side until chest x-ray shows no pneumothorax.

II. **Pulmonary Tubes**
   A. **Endotracheal Tubes:** Verify that the tube is located 3 cm below the vocal cords and 4-5 cm above the carina; the tip should be located at the level of aortic arch.
   B. **Tracheostomy:** Verify by that the tube is located half the distance from the stoma to the carina; the tube should be parallel to the long axis of the trachea. The tube should be approximately 2/3 of width of trachea, and the cuff should not cause bulging of the trachea walls. Check for subcutaneous air in the neck tissue and for mediastinal widening secondary to air leakage.
   C. **Chest Tubes:** A chest tube for pneumothorax drainage should be located at the mid-clavicular line at the level of the third intercostal space. To drain a pulmonary effusion, the tube should be located at the mid to posterior axillary line at the level of the seventh intercostal space. Obtain a chest x-ray to determine position of diaphragm before insertion of chest tube if time permits.
   D. **Mechanical Ventilation:** Obtain a chest x-ray to rule out pneumothorax, subcutaneous emphysema, or pneumomediastinum. Infiltrates may diminish or disappear due to increased aeration of the affected lung lobe.

III. **Gastrointestinal Tubes**
   A. **Nasogastric Tubes:** Verify that the tube is in the stomach and not coiled in the esophagus or trachea. The tip of the tube should be in the gastric antrum and should not be near gastroesophageal junction. Insufflate air and listen over the epigastrium to help confirm tube placement.

## Blood Component Therapy

I. **Crystalloids Solutions:** Normal saline, lactated Ringers solution; used for acute volume replacement. 3 cc crystalloid = 1 cc whole blood.

## II. Colloid Solution Therapy: Indicated for volume expansion.
**A. Albumin (5% or 25%):** Useful for hypovolemia or to induce diuresis with furosemide in hypervolemic, hypoproteinemic patients. Use salt poor albumin in cirrhosis. Hespan is useful for volume expansion and raising osmotic pressure.
**B. Purified Protein Fraction (Plasmanate):** 83% albumin and 17% globulin; indicated for volume expansion.
**C. Hetastarch (Hespan):** Synthetic colloid; 6% hetastarch in saline. Similar indications as for albumin. Maximum dose 1500 cc per 24 hours.

## III. Management of Acute Blood Loss and Red Blood Cell Transfusions
**A.** Control hemorrhage and infuse crystalloids until packed red blood cells are available to replace losses. In trauma, bleeding may require surgical control.
**B.** If crystalloids fail to produce hemodynamic stability after more than 2 liters have been administered, give red blood cells.
**C.** If volume replacement and hemostasis stabilize hemodynamic status, wait for formal type and cross match of blood. In exigent bleeding, administer O negative, low titer blood or type specific (ABO matched), Rh compatible blood which can be obtained rapidly and should be used. Use only in absolute emergency.

## IV. Guidelines for Blood Transfusion in Anemia
Consider blood transfusion when hemoglobin is less than 8.0 and hematocrit is less than 24%. If the patient has symptoms of anemia such as chest pain, dyspnea, poor wound healing, mental status changes, earlier transfusion should be provided.

## V. Blood Component Products
**A. Packed Red Blood Cells (PRBC's):** Each unit provides 250 cc of volume, and each unit should raise hemoglobin by 1 gm/dL and hematocrit by 3%.
**B. Platelets:** Indicated for bleeding due to thrombocytopenia or thrombopathy. Each unit should raise platelet count by 5,000-10,000. Usually transfused 8-10 units at a time. Consider platelet transfusion after 8-10 units of blood replacement.
**C. Fresh Frozen Plasma (FFP):** Used for bleeding secondary to liver disease, dilutional coagulopathy (from multiple blood transfusions), coagulation factor deficiencies. Requires ABO typing, but not cross matching. Improvement of PT/PTT usually requires 2-3 units. Use one unit of FFP for every four units of PRBC's.
**D. Autologous Blood:** Patient donates blood within 35 days of surgery; frozen blood can be stored for up to 2 years. Useful in elective orthopedic, cardiac, and peripheral vascular procedures. Check preoperative hematocrit.

# Fluids and Electrolytes

## I. Maintenance Fluid Guidelines
70 kg Male: D5 ½ NS with 20 mEq KCL/liter at 125 mL/hr.

## II. Pediatric Patients
**A.** Use D5 1/4 NS with 20 mEq KCL/liter.
**B.** 24 hour water requirement, Kg Method: For the first 10 kg body weight: 100 mL/kg/day PLUS For the second 10 kg body weight: 50 mL/kg/day

PLUS For weight above 20 kg: 20 mL/kg/day. Divide by 24 hours to determine hourly rate.

III. **Specific Replacement Fluids of Specific Losses**
   A. **Gastric (nasogastric tube, emesis):** D5 1/2 NS with 20 mEq/liter KCL, replace equal volume of lost fluid q6h.
   B. **Diarrhea:** D5LR with 15 mEq/liter KCL. Provide approximately 1 liter replacement for each 1 kg or 2.2 lb of lost body weight, bicarbonate 45 mEq (1/2 amp) per liter may be added.
   C. **Bile:** D5LR with 25 mEq/liter (1/2 amp) of bicarbonate.
   D. **Pancreatic:** D5LR with 50 mEq/liter (1 amp) bicarbonate.
   E. If unusual volume of fluid loss, send aliquot to lab for electrolyte determination.

# Evaluation of Postoperative Fever

I. **Clinical Evaluation**
   A. **History:** Fever ≥ 100.4-101 F. Determine how many days since operation.
   B. **Differential Diagnosis:** Pneumonia, urinary tract infection, thrombophlebitis, wound infection, drug reaction.
   C. Dysuria, abdominal pain, calf pain. Cough, sputum, headache, stiff neck, joint or back pain.
   D. IV catheter infection (central or peripheral) is an important source of postoperative sepsis.
   E. **Fever Pattern:** Check previous day for fever patterns; spiking fevers indicate abscesses. Continual fevers indicate vascular involvement such as infected prosthetic grafts or septic phlebitis from central IV lines.
   F. Chills or rigors indicate bacteremia, and are usually not associated with atelectasis or drug fevers.
   G. Check for fevers prior to the operation. IV or Foley catheter; alcohol use. Allergies; recent WBC count and differential.

II. **Physical Exam**
   A. **General:** Temperature. Fever curve, tachycardia, hypotension. Examine wound and all vascular access sites carefully.
   B. **HEENT:** Pharyngeal erythema, neck rigidity.
   C. **Chest:** Rhonchi, crackles, dullness to percussion (pneumonia), murmurs (endocarditis).
   D. **Abdomen:** Masses, liver tenderness, Murphy's sign (right upper quadrant tenderness with inspiration, cholecystitis); ascites. Costovertebral angle or suprapubic tenderness.
   E. **Extremities:** Infected decubitus ulcers or wounds; IV catheter tenderness (phlebitis); calf tenderness, joint tenderness (septic arthritis). Cellulitis, furuncles, abscesses. Perirectal abscess, buttock abscess from injections.
   F. **Genitourinary:** Prostate tenderness; rectal flocculence. Cervical discharge, cervical motion tenderness; adnexal tenderness.

III. **Laboratory Evaluation:** CBC, blood C&S X 2, SMA7, UA, urine C&S; lumbar puncture; blood, urine, sputum, wound cultures; chest X-ray.

IV. **Differential Diagnosis**
   A. Wound infection, abscesses, intra-abdominal abscess, atelectasis, drug fever, pulmonary emboli, pancreatitis, alcohol withdrawal, deep vein thrombosis, tuberculosis, cystitis, pyelonephritis, osteomyelitis; IV catheter

phlebitis, sinusitis, otitis media, upper respiratory infection, pelvic infection, cellulitis; hepatitis, infected decubitus ulcer, peritonitis, endocarditis, diverticulitis, cholangitis, carcinomas.
- B. **Medications Associated with Fever:** H2 blockers, penicillins, phenytoin, sulfonamides.
- V. **Antibiotics:** Antibiotic therapy should be initiated immediately if there is any possibility of infection.

# Sepsis

- I. **Pathophysiology**
    - A. Gram-negative organisms are responsible for 50-80% of all cases of septic shock, while 6-24% of cases result from gram-positive organisms. Parasitic infections, disseminated tuberculosis, and systemic fungal disease are less common causes of sepsis.
    - B. The most common source of gram-negative infection is the genitourinary system.
    - C. **Systemic Inflammatory Response Syndromes (SIRS)** is defined as Two or more of the following:
        1. Temperature >38 degrees C or <36 degrees C
        2. Heart rate >90 beats/min
        3. Respiratory rate >20 breaths/min
        4. White blood cell count >12,000 or <4,000 or >10% bands
    - D. SIRS is commonly caused by infection, but a number of other conditions can cause this syndrome (ie, trauma, burns, pancreatitis).
    - E. **Sepsis** consists of SIRS plus a documented infection.
    - F. **Severe Sepsis** consists of sepsis plus end-organ dysfunction (eg, hypoxemia, elevated lactate, oliguria, altered mentation).
    - G. **Septic Shock** is defined as sepsis with hypotension despite fluid resuscitation plus hypoperfusion abnormalities.
    - H. **Refractory Shock** is defined as septic shock that lasts more than 1 hour and does not respond to fluid or pressors.
- II. **Clinical and Laboratory Manifestations of Sepsis**
    - A. The earliest signs of sepsis are tachypnea, respiratory alkalosis, and a moderate hyperdynamic state (increased cardiac output and diminished systemic vascular resistance [SVR]) with little change in blood pressure.
    - B. As septic shock progresses, hypotension results from a decrease in SVR which may overwhelm the increase in cardiac output. Hypoperfusion is manifested by oliguria, hypoxemia, and lactic acidosis.
    - C. **Fever** is common, although, 15% of patients may be hypothermic at onset of bacteremia, and 5% never have a temperature above 99.6° F.
    - D. **Hematologic Abnormalities**
        1. Disseminated intravascular coagulopathy (DIC) occurs in 10% of septic patients, but only 2-3% have significant bleeding.
        2. This syndrome can appear as hemorrhage, thrombosis, or microangiopathic hemolysis.
        3. Laboratory findings include decreased platelets and fibrinogen with elevated prothrombin time, partial thromboplastin time, and fibrin degradation products.
        4. **Neutrophilic leukocytosis** with many band forms (left shift) is the most common hematologic change seen in sepsis. Neutropenia is

much less common.

### E. Renal Effects
1. The effect of sepsis on renal function ranges from minimal proteinuria to acute tubular necrosis, renal failure, and death.
2. Diminished effective circulating volume and hypotension cause renal hypoperfusion with ischemia resulting in acute tubular necrosis.

### F. Adult Respiratory Distress Syndrome
1. Sepsis is the most frequent predisposing factor of ARDS. It is characterized by increased pulmonary capillary permeability resulting in increased extravascular lung water, a widening of the alveolar-arterial 02 gradient, and hypoxemia ($PO_2$ <65 mm Hg), despite efforts at increased oxygenation (40-50% $O_2$ by mask).

### G. Cutaneous Manifestations
1. **Ecthyma gangrenosum** is the most notable finding, but vesicles, bullae, petechiae, diffuse erythema can occur.
2. Skin lesions should be aspirated, cultured and gram-stained.

## III. Clinical Evaluation of Sepsis
### A. Blood Cultures.
Two to three sets of blood cultures from separate sites are adequate to detect most cases of bacteremia.
### B. Gram Strain of Buffy Coat
is positive in up to 50% of cases.
### C.
Hyperglycemia often occurs and may require insulin.
### D.
Hyperbilirubinemia, minimal transaminase, and alkaline phosphatase elevations are often present because of intrahepatic cholestasis.

## Laboratory Tests for Serious Infections

| | |
|---|---|
| Complete blood count, including leukocyte differential and platelet count<br>Electrolytes<br>Arterial blood gases<br>Blood urea nitrogen and creatinine<br>Urinalysis<br>INR, partial thromboplastin time, fibrinogen<br>Serum lactate | Cultures with antibiotic sensitivities<br>  Blood<br>  Urine<br>  Endometrium (if endometritis suspected)<br>  Amniotic fluid (if chorioamnionitis suspected)<br>  Wound<br>  Other sites (eg, sputum, drains)<br>Chest X-ray<br>Adjunctive imaging studies (eg, computed tomography, magnetic resonance imaging, abdominal X-ray) |

## IV. Clinical Management of Sepsis
### A. Resuscitation
1. Fluid resuscitation can begin with immediate rapid infusion of crystalloid (1-2 L of lactated Ringer's or normal saline over 15-20 minutes). Further hemodynamic therapy should be guided by pulmonary artery catheter pressures.
2. After the initial fluid bolus, crystalloid solution may be administered at 10 mL/min for 15 minutes. If the PCWP does not increase by 3 mm Hg, the 1 liter fluid bolus is repeated. Optimal PCWP is in the range of 10-15 mm Hg.
3. Significant hemodilution may result from the large volumes of fluids; a hemoglobin level of at least 10 g/dL should be maintained.

## B. Oxygenation and Ventilation

1. The increased work of breathing and respiratory muscle fatigue during sepsis often necessitates ventilatory support.
2. In the patient with sepsis, oxygen therapy should be started if there is arterial hypoxemia: Oxygen saturation less than 90-92%, or $pAO_2$ less than 60 mm Hg.
3. Positive end-expiratory pressure is frequently necessary to maintain oxygenation.

## C. Vasoactive Drugs

1. Vasoactive drugs are frequently required because of myocardial depression and persistent hypotension.
2. **Dopamine** is the initial drug of choice for improving cardiac function and blood pressure in septic shock. At low doses (1-3 mcg/kg/min), dopamine reacts with dopaminergic receptors, causing vasodilation and increased blood flow in the renal vasculature. At intermediate doses (5-10 mcg/kg/min), beta-adrenergic effects are predominant, which increase myocardial contractility. At high doses (10-20 mcg/kg/min), alpha-adrenergic vasoconstriction is seen including the renal arteries.
3. If dopamine does not adequately support blood pressure, differentiate whether there is persistent vasodilation (blood pressure less than 80 mm Hg with SVR less than 1,400 dynes/s/cm$^3$) or depressed left ventricular function (low left ventricular stroke work index). If depressed myocardium is the major cause, inotropic therapy with dobutamine should be started; if persistent vasodilation is the problem, a peripheral vasoconstrictor (norepinephrine) should be used.

## Commonly Used Vasoactive and Inotropic Drugs

| Agent | Dosage |
|---|---|
| Dopamine | **Renal Perfusion Dose:** 1-3 mcg/kg/min (dopaminergic range)<br>**Cardiac Inotropic Dose:** 5-10 mcg/kg/min (beta-adrenergic)<br>**Vasoconstricting Dose:** 10-20 mcg/kg/min (alpha-adrenergic) |
| Dobutamine | **Inotropic:** 5-10 mcg/kg/min<br>**Vasodilator:** 15-20 mcg/kg/min |
| Norepinephrine | 2-8 mcg/min |
| Phenylephrine | 20-200 mcg/min |
| Epinephrine | 1-8 mcg/min |

## D. Treatment of Infection

1. The choice of drugs should be based on the probable source of infection, gram-stained smears of clinical specimens, the immune status of the patient, and local patterns of bacterial resistance.
2. Aggressive dosing of antibiotics is recommended.
3. **Sepsis.** For initial treatment of life-threatening sepsis in adults, a third-generation cephalosporin (cefotaxime, ceftizoxime), ticarcillin/clavulanic acid or imipenem, each together with an

aminoglycoside (gentamicin, tobramycin, or amikacin) is recommended.
4. **Methicillin-Resistant Staphylococci.** When MRSA is suspected, treatment with vancomycin (with gentamicin) is recommended.
5. **Intra-Abdominal or Pelvic Infections** are likely to involve anaerobes; treatment should include either ticarcillin/clavulanic acid, ampicillin/sulbactam, piperacillin/tazobactam, imipenem, cefoxitin or cefotetan, each with an aminoglycoside or, alternatively, metronidazole or clindamycin, together with an aminoglycoside and ampicillin is necessary.
6. **Biliary Tract Infections:** When the source of bacteremia is thought to be in the biliary tract, cefoperazone, piperacillin plus metronidazole, piperacillin/tazobactam, or ampicillin/sulbactam, each with an aminoglycoside, should be used.
7. **Antibiotic-Resistant Gram-Negative Bacilli.** In some hospitals, gram-negative bacilli have become resistant to aminoglycosides, third-generation cephalosporins and aztreonam; these strains may be susceptible to imipenem or ciprofloxacin.
8. **Multiple-Antibiotic-Resistant Enterococci**
   a. Many enterococcal strains are now resistant to ampicillin, gentamicin, and vancomycin. A few vancomycin-resistant enterococci are susceptible to teicoplanin (Targocid). Some strains are susceptible to chloramphenicol, doxycycline, or fluoroquinolones.
   b. Quinupristin/dalfopristin (Synercid) (investigational) is active against most strains of multiple-drug-resistant Enterococcus.
   c. Polymicrobial surgical infections that include antibiotic-resistant enterococci may respond to antibiotics aimed at the other organisms.
9. **Dosages of Antibiotics Used in Sepsis**
   a. Cefotaxime (Claforan) 2 gm q4-6h.
   b. Ceftizoxime (Cefizox) 2 gm IV q8h.
   c. Cefoxitin (Mefoxin) 2 gms q6-8h.
   d. Cefotetan (Cefotan) 2 gms IV q12h.
   e. Ceftazidime (Fortaz) 2 g IV q8h.
   f. Ticarcillin/clavulanate (Timentin) 3.1 gm IV q4-6h (200-300 mg/kg/d).
   g. Ampicillin/Sulbactam (Unasyn) 3.0 gm IV q6h.
   h. Piperacillin/tazobactam (Zosyn) 3.375-4.5 gm IV q6h.
   i. Piperacillin, ticarcillin, mezlocillin 3 gms IV q4-6h.
   j. Meropenem (Merrem) 1 gm IV q8h.
   k. Gentamicin, tobramycin 5 mg/kg IV qd; or 100-120 mg (1.5-2 mg/kg) IV, then 80 mg IV q8h (3-5 mg/kg/d).
   l. Amikacin (Amikin) 7.5 mg/kg IV loading dose; then 5 mg/kg IV q8h.
   m. Vancomycin 1 gm IV q12h.
   n. Ofloxacin (Floxin) 400 mg IV q12h.
   o. Aztreonam (Azactam) 1-2 gm IV q6-8h; max 8 g/day.
   p. Metronidazole (Flagyl) 500 mg IV q6-8h.
   q. Clindamycin 600-900 IV q8h (15-30 mg/kg/d).
E. The third-generation cephalosporins (ceftazidime, ceftizoxime, cefotaxime) or meropenem can be used to treat sepsis caused by many

strains of gram-negative bacilli.
- **F.** Ceftazidime has less activity against gram-positive cocci. Cephalosporins other than ceftazidime and cefoperazone have limited activity against Pseudomonas aeruginosa.
- **G.** Imipenem and aztreonam are active against most strains of P. aeruginosa, and imipenem is active against anaerobes.
- **H.** Aztreonam is active against aerobic gram-negative bacilli, but has poor activity against gram-positive bacteria and anaerobes.

# Enteral Nutrition

## I. Enteral Feeding

- **A. General Measures:** Daily weights, I&O. Head of bed at 30° while enteral feeding and 2 hours after completion. Confirm placement of tube with an X-ray and by instillation of air in tube while auscultating over epigastrium. Do not give enteral feedings in postoperative patients until ileus resolved and gastric emptying is satisfactory. Always check stomach residual fluid before NG feeding. Record bowel movements. Nutrition consult may be useful.
- **B. Enteral Bolus Feeding:** Give 50-100 mL of enteral solution (eg: Osmolite) q3h initially. Increase amount in 50 mL steps to max of 250-300 mL q3-4h; 30 kcal of nonprotein calories/d and 1.5 gm protein/kg/d. Before each feeding measure residual volume, and delay feeding by 1h if >100 mL. Flush tube with 100 cc of water after each bolus.
- **C. Continuous Enteral Infusion** - Initial enteral solution (Osmolite) 30 mL/hr. Measure residual volume q1h x 12h, then tid; hold feeding for 1h if 100 mL. Increase rate by 25-50 mL/hr at 24 hr intervals as tolerated until final rate of 50-100 mL/hr as tolerated. 3 Tablespoons of protein powder (Promix) may be added to each 500 cc of solution. Flush tube with 100 cc water q8h. Do not advance enteral feeding if diarrhea develops.
- **D. Symptomatic Medications**
  1. Loperamide (Imodium) 2-4 mg PO/J-tube q6h, max 16 mg/d prn OR
  2. Diphenoxylate/atropine (Lomotil) 1-2 tabs or 5-10 mL (2.5 mg/5 mLs) PO/J-tube q4-6h prn, max 12 tabs/d
  3. Kaopectate 30 cc PO or in J-tube q8h.

# Parenteral Nutrition

## I. Central Parenteral Nutrition

- **Indications for TPN:** Severe malnutrition (albumin <3.0 or >10% loss of body weight), prolonged postoperative ileus, intestinal fistula, pancreatitis. Infuse 40-50 mL/h of amino acid-dextrose solution in the first 24h; increase daily by 40 mL/hr increments until providing 1.3-2 times the basal energy requirement and 1.2-1.7 gm protein/kg/d (formula in appendix).

# 20 Parenteral Nutrition

## Standard solution (1 liter) (adjust TPN as needed to maintain normal electrolytes)

| | |
|---|---|
| Amino Acid (Aminosyn) 7-10% | 500 mL |
| Dextrose 40-70% | 500 mL |
| Sodium | 35 mEq |
| Potassium | 36 mEq |
| Chloride | 35 mEq |
| Calcium | 4.5 mEq |
| Phosphate | 9 mMol |
| Magnesium | 8.0 mEq |
| Acetate | 82-104 mEq |
| Multi-Trace Element Formula | 1 mL/d |
| Regular Insulin (if indicated) | 10-60 U/L |
| Multivitamin(12) (2 amp) | 10 mL/d |
| Vitamin K (in solution, SQ, IM) | 10 mg/week |
| Vitamin B12 | 1000 mcg/week |

Intralipid 20%, 500 mL/d intravenous piggyback, infused in parallel with standard solution at 1 mL/min x 15 min; if no adverse reactions, increase to 100 mL/hr. Serum triglyceride 6h after infusion (maintain <200 mg/dL).

- **A. Cyclic TPN** 12h night schedule; Taper continuous infusion in morning by reducing rate to half original rate for 1 hour. Further reduce rate by half for an additional hr; then discontinue. Restart TPN in afternoon. Taper in beginning and end of cycle. Final rate of 185 mL/hr for 12h and 1 hour of taper at each end for total of 2000 mL.
- **B. Special Medications**
  1. Metoclopramide (Reglan) 10-20 mg PO, IM, IV, or in J tube q6h.
  2. Cimetidine 300 mg PO tid-qid or 37.5-100 mg/h IV or 300 mg IV q6-8h or in TPN **OR**
  3. Ranitidine 50 mg IV q6-8h or 150 mg PO bid or in TPN.
  4. Insulin sliding scale.

## II. Peripheral Parenteral Supplementation

- **A.** 3% amino acid sln (ProCalamine) up to 3 L/d at 125 cc/h **OR**
- **B.** Combine 500 mL Amino acid solution (7% or 10%) (Aminosyn) and 500 mL of 20% dextrose and electrolyte additive, and infuse at up to 100 cc/hr in parallel with: Intralipid 10% or 20% at 1 mL/min for 15 min (test dose); if no adverse reactions, infuse 500 mL/d at up to 100 mL/hr.
  1. Draw blood 6h after end of infusion for triglycerides.
- **C. Laboratory Evaluation**
  1. **Baseline** - draw all labs below. CXR, plain film for tube placement
  2. **Daily Labs** - SMA7, osmolality, CBC, cholesterol, triglyceride (6 h after infusion).
  3. **Weekly Labs** - Cal, phosphorous, SMA-12
  4. **Weekly Labs When Indicated** - Protein, Mg, iron, TIBC, transferrin, PT/PTT, zinc, copper, B12, Folate, 24h urine nitrogen and creatinine. Pre-albumin, retinol-binding protein.

# Central Venous Catheterization

I. **Indications for Central Venous Catheter Cannulation:** Monitoring of central venous pressures in shock or heart failure; management of fluid status; administration of total parenteral nutrition. Also used as route for temporary dialysis access and for prolonged antimicrobial or chemotherapy.

II. **Location of Catheterization Site**
   A. The internal jugular approach is contraindicated in patients with a carotid bruit, stenosis, or aneurysm.
   B. Subclavian approach has increased risk in patients with emphysema or bullae.
   C. The external jugular or internal jugular approach by direct cut-down may be preferable in patients with coagulopathy or thrombocytopenia.
   D. In patients with a chest tube already in place, the catheter should usually be placed on the side with the chest tube.

III. **Technique of Insertion for External Jugular Vein**
   A. The external jugular vein courses from angle of mandible to behind the middle of clavicle, where it joins with the subclavian vein. Place patient in Trendelenburg's position, and apply digital pressure to the external jugular vein above clavicle to distend vein. Cleanse skin with Betadine iodine solution using sterile technique; inject 1% lidocaine to produce a skin weal.
   B. With an 18-gauge thin wall needle, advance the needle into the vein. Then pass a J-guide wire through the needle; the wire should advance without resistance. Remove the needle, maintaining control over the guide wire at all times. Nick the skin with a No. 11 scalpel blade.
   C. With guide wire in place, pass the central catheter over the wire, and remove the guide wire after the catheter is in place. Cover catheter hub with a finger to prevent air embolization.
   D. Attach a syringe to the catheter hub, and ensure that there is free backflow of dark venous blood. Attach the catheter to an intravenous infusion at a keep open rate.
   E. Secure the catheter in place with 2-0 silk suture and tape.
   F. Obtain a CXR to confirm position and rule out pneumothorax.
   G. The catheter should be removed and changed within 3-4 days.

IV. **Internal Jugular Vein Cannulation:** The internal jugular vein is positioned behind the sternocleidomastoid muscle, lateral to the carotid artery. The catheter should be placed at a location at the upper confluence of the two bellies of sternocleidomastoid, at the level of cricoid cartilage.
   A. Place the patient in Trendelenburg's position, and turn the patient's head to the contralateral side.
   B. Choose a location on the right or left. If all other factors are equal (symmetrical lung function, no chest tubes in place), the right side is preferred because of the direct path to the superior vena cava. Prepare the skin with Betadine solution using sterile technique and drape the area. Infiltrate the skin and deeper tissues with 1% lidocaine.
   C. Palpate the carotid artery. Using a 22-gauge scout needle and syringe, direct the needle toward the nipple at a 30 degree angle to the neck. While aspirating, advance the needle until the vein is located and blood back flows into the syringe.
   D. Remove the scout needle and advance an 18-gauge, thin wall, catheter-over-needle with an attached syringe along the same path as the scout

needle. When back flow of blood is noted into syringe, advance the catheter into the vein. Remove the needle and confirm back flow of blood through the catheter and into the syringe. Remove syringe and cover the catheter hub with a finger to prevent air embolization.
   E. With the catheter in position, advance a 0.89 mm x 45 cm guide wire through the catheter. The guide wire should advance easily without resistance.
   F. With the guide wire in position, remove the catheter and use a No. 11 scalpel blade to nick the skin.
   G. Place central vein catheter over the wire, holding the wire secure at all times. Pass the catheter into the vein, and suture the catheter with O silk suture, tape, and connect to IV infusion at a keep open rate.
   H. Obtain a CXR to rule out pneumothorax and confirm position.
V. **Subclavian Vein Cannulation**
   A. The subclavian vein is located in the angle formed by the medial 1/3 of clavicle and the first rib.
   B. Position the patient supine with a rolled towel located longitudinally between the patient's scapulae, and turn the patient's head towards the contralateral side. Prepare the area with Betadine iodine solution, and, using sterile technique, drape the area and infiltrate 1% lidocaine into the skin and tissues.
   C. With a 16-gauge catheter-over-needle with syringe attached, puncture the mid-point of the clavicle until the clavicle bone and needle come in contact.
   D. Then slowly probe down until the needle slips under the clavicle. Advance the needle slowly towards the vein until the needle enters the vein, and a back flow of venous blood enters the syringe. Remove the syringe, and cover the catheter hub with a finger to prevent air embolization.
   E. With the 16-gauge catheter in position, advance a 0.89 mm x 45 cm guide wire through the catheter. The guide wire should advance easily without resistance.
   F. With the guide wire in position, remove the catheter and use a No. 11 scalpel blade to nick the skin.
   G. Pass dilator over the wire.
   H. Place the central line catheter over the wire, holding the wire secure at all times. Pass the catheter into the vein, and suture the catheter with 2-0 silk suture, tape the catheter in place and connect to IV infusion.
   I. Obtain a CXR to confirm position and rule out pneumothorax.

# Pulmonary Artery Catheterization

1. Cannulate a vein using the technique above, such as the subclavian vein or internal jugular.
2. Advance a guide wire through the cannula, and remove the cannula. Nick the skin with number 11 scalpel blade adjacent to the guide wire, and pass a number 8 French introducer over the wire into the vein. Connect introducer to an IV fluid infusion at a keep open rate, and suture introducer in place with 2-0 silk.
3. Pass the proximal end of the pulmonary artery catheter (Swan Ganz) to an assistant for connection to a continuous flush transducer system.

4. Flush the distal and proximal ports with heparin solution, removing all bubbles, and check balloon integrity by inflating 2 cc of air. Check pressure transducer response by moving the distal tip quickly.
5. Pass the catheter through the introducer into the vein, then inflate the balloon, and advance the catheter until the balloon is in or near the right atrium.
6. As a general guideline, the correct distance to the entrance of the right atrium is determined from the site of insertion:
   Right antecubital fossa: 35-40 cm
   Left antecubital fossa: 45-50 cm.
   Right internal jugular vein: 10-15 cm.
   Subclavian vein: 10 cm.
   Femoral vein: 35-45 cm.
7. Run a continuous monitoring strip to record pressures as the PA catheter is advanced.
8. Advance the balloon, inflated with 0.8-1.0 cc of air, while monitoring pressures and wave forms. Advance the catheter through the right ventricle into the main pulmonary artery until the catheter enters a distal branch of the pulmonary artery and is stopped by impaction (as evidenced by a pulmonary wedge pressure wave form).
9. Do not advance catheter with balloon deflated, and do not withdraw the catheter with the balloon inflated. After placement, obtain a chest X-ray to insure that the tip of catheter is no farther than 3-5 cm from midline, and no pneumothorax is present.

# Normal Pulmonary Artery Catheter Values

| | |
|---|---|
| Right atrial pressure | 1-7 mm Hg |
|     RVP Systolic | 15-25 mm Hg |
|     RVP Diastolic | 8-15 mm Hg |
| | |
| Pulmonary artery pressure | |
|     PAP Systolic | 15-25 mm Hg |
|     PAP Diastolic | 8-15 mm Hg |
|     PAP Mean | 10-20 mm Hg |
| | |
| PCWP | 6-12 mm Hg |
| | |
| Cardiac Output | 3.5-5.5 L/min |
| Cardiac Index | 2.0-3.2 L/min/m$^2$ |
| Systemic Vascular Resistance | 800-1200 dyne/sec/cm$^2$ |

# Venous Cutdown

### Procedures

1. Obtain a prepackaged cutdown tray, or a minor procedure tray and instrument tray with a silk suture (3-0, 4-0) and a catheter. This procedure will require gloves, sterile towels/drapes, 4 x 4 gauze sponges, povidone-iodine solution, 5 cc syringe, 25 gauge needle, 1% lidocaine with epinephrine, adhesive tape, scissors, needle holder, hemostat, scalpel and blade. suture. Adequate

lighting and assistance should be available before beginning procedure.
2. Apply a tourniquet proximal to the site, and identify the vein. Prep the skin with povidone-iodine solution and drape area. Infiltrate the skin with 1% lidocaine, then incise the skin transversely.
3. Spread the incision long-wise in the direction of the vein with a hemostat and dissect any adherent tissue from the vein. Lift the vein and pass two chromic or silk ties (3-0 or 4-0) behind the vein.
4. Tie off the distal suture, using the upper tie for traction. Make a transverse nick in the vein. If necessary, use a catheter introducer to hold the lumen of the vein open.
5. Make a small stab incision in the skin distal to the main skin incision, and insert a plastic catheter or IV cannula through the incision, then insert it into vein. Tie the proximal suture, and attach IV fluid, release the tourniquet. Suture skin with silk or nylon, and apply dressing.

## Arterial Line Placement

**Procedure**
1. Obtain a 20 gauge, 1 1/2-2 inch catheter-over-needle assembly (Angiocath), arterial line setup (transducer, tubing, pressure bag containing heparinized saline), armboard, sterile dressing, 1% lidocaine, 3 cc syringe, 25 gauge needle, 3-0 silk.
2. The radial artery is used. Use the Allen Test to verify patency of the radial artery and adequacy of ulnar artery collaterals. Place the extremity on an armboard with a gauze roll behind the wrist to maintain hyperextension.
3. Prep with povidone-iodine and drape; infiltrate 1% lidocaine using a 25 gauge needle. Choose a site where the artery is most superficial and as distal as possible on the wrist.
4. Palpate the artery with the left hand, and use other hand to advance a 20 gauge catheter-over-needle into the artery at a 30 degree angle to the skin. When a flash of blood is seen, hold the needle in place and advance the catheter into the artery; occlude the artery with manual pressure while the pressure tubing is connected.
5. If a needle and guide-wire kits is used, advance the guide wire into the artery, and pass the catheter over the guide-wire.
6. Suture catheter in place with 3-0 silk and apply dressing.

## Cricothyrotomy

### I. Needle Cricothyrotomy
**A.** Obtain a 12-14 gauge, catheter-over-needle (Angiocath or Jelco), 6-12 mL syringe, 3 mm pediatric endotracheal tube adapter, oxygen tubing, and a high flow oxygen source.
**B.** Locate the cricothyroid membrane (notch between the thyroid cartilage and cricoid cartilage).
**C.** Cleanse the neck area with povidone-iodine solution, and inject 2% lidocaine with epinephrine (if the patient is awake).
**D.** With a 12 or 14 gauge, catheter-over-needle assembly on the syringe, advance needle through the cricothyroid membrane at a 45 degree

angle directed inferiorly. Apply back pressure on the syringe until air is aspirated.
- E. Advance the catheter and remove the needle, then attach the hub to a 3 mm endotracheal tube adapter connected to oxygen tubing.
- F. Administer oxygen at 15 liters per minute for 1-2 seconds on, then 4 seconds off; control air flow by using a Y-connector or a hole in the side of the tubing.
- G. The needle cricothyrotomy should be replaced with oral endotracheal intubation as soon as feasible. A needle cricothyrotomy should not be used for more than 45 minutes, since exhalation of $CO_2$ is inadequate.

## II. Surgical Cricothyrotomy

- A. Obtain a #5-#7 tracheostomy tube; tracheostomy tube adapter to connect to bag-mask ventilator; povidone-iodine solution, sterile gauze pads, scalpel handle, and hemostat.
- B. Clean the neck area with providone-iodine.
- C. Locate the thyroid and cricoid cartilages; the cricothyroid membrane extends between these two cartilages.
- D. Infiltrate the overlying skin with 2% lidocaine with epinephrine if the patient is awake.
- E. Stabilize the thyroid cartilage with the left hand, and make a transverse incision through the skin and subcutaneous tissues overlying the cricothyroid membrane, avoiding the large vessels that are located laterally.
- F. Make a stab incision inferiorly in the cricothyroid membrane with the point of the blade.
- G. Insert the knife handle, and rotate the handle 90 degrees to open the hole; or use a hemostat to dilate the opening.
- H. Gently insert the tube and secure with tape.
- I. The surgical cricothyrotomy should be replaced with a formal tracheostomy within a few hours.

**26 Cricothyrotomy**

# *Trauma*

Charles F. Chandler, M.D.

## Management of the Trauma Patient

I. **Primary Survey of the Trauma Patient:** Assess airway, breathing, and circulation (ABC's).
   - A = Airway maintenance with cervical spine stabilization.
   - B = Assess breathing, administer assisted ventilations if required; rule out tension pneumothorax.
   - C = Assess circulation and control hemorrhage.
   - D = Assess disability and neurologic status.
   - E = Exposure; completely undress patient; prevent hypothermia.

II. **Resuscitation Phase**
   - A. Assess adequacy of airway and ventilation, evaluate control of hemorrhage, initiate fluid resuscitation. Early intubation is recommended if the airway is compromised (eg orofacial trauma), or if there is severe closed head injury or hemorrhagic shock.
   - B. Place a minimum of two large bore IVs. Blood should be drawn for type and cross, hemoglobin or hematocrit, and electrolytes. Initial and follow-up hemoglobin or spun hematocrit should be rapidly determined in the emergency department.
   - C. Administer crystalloids. Initial fluid bolus of 1-2 liters of Ringer's lactate (20 cc/kg in pediatric patients).
   - D. Evaluate for improvement in blood pressure, decrease in pulse rate, improved skin circulation and capillary refill, increase in urine output, and improved mental status.
   - E. If there has been significant hemorrhage, or there has been failure to restore systolic pressure >100mm Hg with crystalloid, transfuse blood.

III. **Ongoing Assessment and Treatment**
   - A. **Administer cross matched,** type-specific, cross matched type O negative blood if patient is unstable.
   - B. **Manage coagulopathy** with empiric administration of fresh frozen plasma, 1 unit FFP for every 4 units of packed red blood cells. Transfuse 10 units platelets per 6 units PRBC. If rapid administration of more than 4 units PRBC, consider calcium gluconate. Avoid hypothermia.
   - C. **Place a nasogastric tube** for decompression of the stomach, and place a Foley catheter to evaluate urine output (caution if facial fracture or unstable cervical spine).
   - D. **Monitor adequacy** of resuscitation, looking for improvement in physiologic parameters such as heart rate, systolic pressure, ventilatory rate, distal perfusion and capillary refill, pulse oximetry.
   - E. **Reassess ABC's** prior to beginning secondary survey.

IV. **Secondary Survey**
   - A. Obtain an abrieviated history including allergies, medications, past illness, Last meal, Event/mechanism= AMPLE history.
   - B. Evaluate the completely undressed patient, front and back and from head to toe, and thoroughly evaluate each system (head and neck, chest,

abdomen, perineum, musculo-skeletal, vascular, neurologic). Check the patient's Glasgow coma scale (GCS) score.
- C. Obtain appropriate X-rays (chest, cervical spine, pelvis) and other procedures (peritoneal lavage, CT scan). Do not send an unstable patient to the radiology department.
- D. **Laboratory Studies:** Send type and cross for 6 units or more of packed red blood cells; complete blood count, platelet count, electrolytes, creatinine, BUN, glucose, calcium, PT/PTT; ethanol level, pregnancy test, arterial blood gases; UA, urine and serum toxicology screens. Liver function tests, amylase.
- E. **Re-evaluation:** constantly re-evaluate for current status/response to therapy.

## V. Definitive Care Phase

- A. After preliminary identification of injuries, begin definitive care management of life threatening emergencies and obtaining urgently required studies.
- B. Reassessment and simultaneous treatment should continue. The most immediate life threatening problems should be treated first: ABC's followed by abdominal trauma; neurologic or head trauma; massive blood loss via pelvic or extremity fractures.

# Abdominal Trauma

- A. Maintain airway, breathing, and circulatory support. Rapid exsanguinating injuries take precedence over other injuries, including head injuries.
- B. **Initial Stabilization:** Control external bleeding with direct external pressure.
- C. Place two number 14 or 16 gauge intravenous lines, type and cross for packed blood cells.
- D. In an emergency (with insufficient time to cross match), give type O-negative blood.
- E. For hypotensive patients, give an initial fluid challenge of 2 L of Ringer's lactate solution over 5-10 min or 20 mL/kg in children over 5-10 min.
- F. **Assess response to initial fluid challenge** by checking blood pressure and heart rate.
- G. **Patients who respond with only a transient increase** in blood pressure should be rechallenged with Ringer's lactate or blood transfusion; blood loss may be continuing.
- H. Patients who have no response to initial fluid challenge may have either extensive blood loss or continued bleeding, and must be given rapid blood transfusion. The site of bleeding must be identified (chest, abdomen, extremities, pelvis) and surgical intervention should be initiated. Other causes of hypotension include tension pneumothorax and cardiac tamponade.
- I. **Manage coagulopathy** with empiric administration of fresh frozen plasma, 1 unit FFP for every 4 units of packed red blood cells. Transfuse 10 units platelets per 6 units PRBC.
- J. Keep the patient, ventilator circuit, and infused fluids warmed. Hypothermia often contributes to coagulopathy. Consider calcium infusion if rapid infusion of greater than 4 U PRBC.
- K. **If peritoneal or visceral penetration is suspected**, broad spectrum

beta-lactam (cefoxitin, cefotetan, Timentin or Zosyn) antibiotic coverage is necessary, but patient should be taken immediately to the operating room. Continue for 48 hours if bowel injury.

# Penetrating Abdominal Trauma

### I. Gun Shot Wounds
   A. All abdominal gun shot wounds require exploratory laparotomy.
   B. Tangential wounds that do not penetrate the peritoneal cavity may be assessed by peritoneal lavage or laparoscopy if wound is located on the anterior abdominal wall.

### II. Stab Wounds and Other Penetrating Abdominal Trauma
   A. Exploratory laparotomy is required if acute abdomen or signs of peritoneal injury, shock, hypotension, upper or lower GI bleeding, evisceration or pneumoperitoneum.
   B. If patient is stable and the abdominal fascia is involved, or penetrated on local exploration, perform diagnostic peritoneal lavage. If lavage is positive, perform exploratory laparotomy. (RBC >1000/mL, WBC >50). The threshold for acceptable cell count is much lower after penetrating abdominal injuries than after blunt abdominal trauma.
   C. Consider tetanus prophylaxis if indicated.

### III. Stab Wounds and Other Sharp Trauma With No Involvement or Penetration of Fascia
   A. These patients should be observed for 24 hours, and local wound care and antibiotics should be administered.
   B. Consider tetanus prophylaxis if indicated.

# Blunt Abdominal Trauma

### I. If Acute Abdomen or Pneumoperitoneum On X-ray:
Perform exploratory laparotomy.

### II. If Non-Acute Abdomen
   A. Perform diagnostic peritoneal lavage or CT scan if possible internal injury.
   B. If patient is not stable (SBP <100, HR >100, decreasing hemoglobin) and abdominal injury is possible, DPL should be done rather than CT scan. If lavage is positive, laporotomy is required.
   C. If a CT scan shows only minor isolated splenic or liver injury, and patient remains stable, the patient may be observed in the ICU. Other injuries mandate laporotomy.
   D. CT scan sensitivity is influenced by the experience of the person reading the scan. CT scan is not sensitive for intestinal or diaphragmatic injury.
   E. In stable patients who do not receive exploratory laporatomy, serial abdominal exams should be performed. If significant findings of tenderness or peritoneal signs, the patient should be evaluated by DPL, CT, or laporotomy.
   F. If significant head injury, intoxication, or distracting injury (eg, multiple rib fractures, pelvic fracture, extremity fracture), the abdominal exam is unreliable, and the patient must be evaluated by DPL or CT scan.
   G. If patient is to undergo a prolonged orthopedic or neurosurgical

procedure, the abdomen should be evaluated with DPL or CT before the procedure; if subdural or epidural hematoma mandates immediate operation, a DPL can be done in the operating room.
- H. DPL will not detect reroperitoneal injuries. Previous abdominal surgery is a relative contraindication to DPL; if DPL is indicated, it should be done by open rather than Seldinger technique. Morbid obesity and advanced cirrhosis are also relative contraindications to DPL.
- I. **Criteria for a Positive Peritoneal Lavage**
    1. Gross blood; red blood cell count >100,000 cells/mm$^3$; white blood cell count >500 cells/mm3.
    2. Presence of food particles, bile, feces, or bacteria on Gram stain.
    3. Exit of lavage fluid via a chest tube or bladder catheter.
    4. Amylase $\geq$20 IU/L; alkaline phosphatase $\geq$3 IU.

# Diagnostic Peritoneal Lavage

- A. Insert a nasogastric tube and Foley catheter to decompress the stomach and the bladder. Restrain or sedate patient if necessary. Prep and drape the periumbilical region with Betadine solution and sterile towels. Select a site above or below umbilicus. If the patient has a pelvic fracture or if pregnant, the site must be above the umbilicus.
- B. Infiltrate the skin and subcutaneous tissue with 1% lidocaine with epinephrine. Incise the skin with a 1-5 cm vertical incision through the subcutaneous tissue down to fascia.
- C. Use a No. 11 scalpel blade to make a stab incision 2-3 mm in length into the fascia.
- D. Apply traction to both sides of fascial incision with towel clips, and have an assistant apply strong upward traction on clips.
- E. Disect bluntly with a small hemostat to peritoneum, then grasp and incise the peritoneum, and introduce a lavage catheter into the pelvis.
- F. Aspirate with a 12 cc syringe. If 6 cc of blood is returned, the lavage should be considered "grossly positive", which mandates an immediate laporotomy. If the aspirate is negative, instill 1 liter of Ringer's lactate or saline from a pressure bag. Periodically agitate the abdomen. When only a small amount of fluid remains in the bag, drop bag to the floor, and drain the fluid by siphon action.
- G. During the procedure keep a sponge packed in the wound and hold catheter in place. After at least 300 cc of fluid have been removed, clamp the tubing and withdraw the catheter.
- H. Close the fascial defect with heavy absorbable suture, and staple the skin.

# Head Trauma

## I. Initial Management of Head Trauma

A. Maintain airway and control cervical spine. Management of Airway Breathing and Circulation must take priority (follow the ABC's of basic cardiac life support).

B. A cervical spine injury should be considered to be present in any patient with multisystem trauma, especially injury involving the area above the clavicles. A normal neurologic examination does not rule out a cervical spine injury.

C. Intravenous resuscitation solutions should be isotonic (lactated Ringers or normal saline).

D. Make an initial assessment of the patient.

E. Perform a mini-neurologic examination as soon as possible and repeat frequently (GCS, pupils, motor/lateralizing signs).

F. If altered mental status, give 50 mLs of 50% dextrose, thiamine 100 mg, and naloxone (Narcan) 0.4-2.0 mg, intravenously.

G. Take a complete history, including the mechanism of injury, past medical history, drug intake.

H. **Glasgow Coma Scale Assessment of Level of Consciousness**

|  | Points |
|---|---|
| **1. Eye Opening** | |
| Spontaneous | 4 |
| To speech | 3 |
| To pain | 2 |
| None | 1 |
| **2. Verbal Response** | |
| Oriented | 5 |
| Confused | 4 |
| Inappropriate words | 3 |
| Incomprehensible sounds | 2 |
| None | 1 |
| **3. Best Motor Response** | |
| Obeys | 6 |
| Localities | 5 |
| Withdraws | 4 |
| Flexion | 3 |
| Extension | 2 |
| None | 1 |

I. Examine skull for clinically detectable depressed, skull fracture; Battle's sign (blood in the ear canal or ecchymosis over mastoid process); Raccoon's eyes (periorbital ecchymosis), rhinorrhea. The patient requires admission if any of these signs are present.

J. Do not place a nasogastric or nasotracheal tube if a cribiform plate fracture is possible.

## II. Secondary Management of Head Trauma

A. All patients need admission and 24 hours of serial neuro-exams unless GCS is 15 and only brief amnesia of events, without loss of consciousness. Such patients may be discharged with instructions if reliable observation ensured.

B. If GCS 14 or less, or if loss of consciousness for more than a few seconds, a head CT scan should be obtained.

C. If the mechanism of injury was significantly violent (rollover of vehicle), or if massive upper torso trauma or any lateralizing neuro deficits, a head CT should be obtained.
   D. **If GCS is less than 8 or if unequal pupils, lateralizing deficits, or Open Head Injury:** There is a high probability of mass effect (subdural, epidural, or intracerebral bleed) or diffuse axonal injury. This patient requires ICU admission after obtaining a CT of head and a neurosurgical consultation. Emergency intubation is required for airway control and hyperventilation to $PCO_2$ 30-32 mm Hg until assessment of intracerebral pressure by head CT and/or ICP monitoring. Intubation is done orotracheally with on-line-traction (do not hyperextend neck).

III. **Ongoing Management of Head Trauma**
   A. Continually reassess ABC's, ECG, systolic, blood pressure, HR, pulse oximeter. Serial Hgb or Hct should be obtained.
   B. Isolated head injuries do not cause hypotension, alternate etiologies must be vigorously sought. Secondary causes of brain injury, such as hypoxia and hypotension should be managed immediately.
   C. Draw blood for CBC, PT, PTT, Chem 18; type and cross matching; toxicology screen, serum osmolarity.
   D. Give stress ulcer prophylaxis with $H_2$-blockers (ranitidine, cimetidine), or sucralfate.
   E. Avoid administration of sedative-hypnotics, narcotics, or neuromuscular blockers unless directed by neurosurgeon.
   F. Control hypothermia aggressively with warming of IV fluids, blood, ventillator circuit, and with warming blankets.
   G. Clean and repair open head wounds.
   H. Give Tetanus prophylaxis with 0.5 cc tetanus toxoid IM, with or without tetanus Ig 250 IU. IM as indicated.
   I. **Antibiotics:** Penetrating head and neck injuries should receive Ancef, abdominal trauma injuries should receive a 2nd generation cephlosporin, open extremity fracture injuries should receive Ancef plus Gentamicin.

# Pneumothorax

I. **Management of Pneumothorax**
   A. **Small Primary Spontaneous Pneumothorax (<10-15%) (no underlying pulmonary disease, isolated injury, and not dyspneic)**
      1. Observe for 24 hours. Treat with high flow oxygen. Repeat exams frequently. Pulse oximeter monitoring.
      2. Repeat chest X-ray in 4 hours. If the pneumothorax does not increase in size, and the patient remains asymptomatic after 24 hours, discharge home. The patient should be instructed to rest and curtail all strenuous activities. Return if increase in dyspnea or recurrence of chest pain.
   B. **Traumatic Pneumothorax associated with a penetrating injury with hemothorax, or traumatic pneumothorax requiring positive pressure ventilation, or with tension pneumothorax**
      1. Give high flow oxygen, and immediately insert a chest tube. Provide aggressive hemodynamic and respiratory resuscitation as indicated.
      2. Do not delay the management of a possible tension pneumothorax until radiographic confirmation; needle thoracostomy may provide

temporizing measure, but insert a chest tube as soon as possible.

## II. Technique of Chest Tube Insertion

- **A.** Place patient in the supine position, with involved side elevated 10-20 degrees, and abduct arm at 90 degrees. The usual site is between the mid-axillary and anterior axillary line at the level of the fourth intercostal space (nipple line). Alternatively, the second or third intercostal space, in the mid-clavicular line may be used for pneumothorax drainage alone (not useful for hemothorax drainage, and should be avoided in the emergency setting).
- **B.** Cleanse skin with Betadine iodine solution and drape the field. Determine the intrathoracic tube distance (lateral chest wall to the apices), and mark length of tube with a clamp.
- **C.** Infiltrate 1% lidocaine into the skin, subcutaneous tissues, intercostal muscles, periosteum, and pleura using a 25-gauge needle. Use a scalpel to make a transverse skin incision, 2 centimeters wide, located over the rib just inferior to the interspace where the tube will penetrate the chest wall.
- **D.** Use a Kelly clamp to bluntly dissect a subcutaneous tunnel from the skin incision, extending just over the superior margin of the rib. Avoid the nerve, artery, and vein located just below each rib.
- **E.** Bluntly dissect over the rib and penetrate the pleura with the clamp, and open the pleura 1 centimeter.
- **F.** With a gloved finger, explore the subcutaneous tunnel, and palpate the lung medially. Exclude possible abdominal penetration, and verify correct location within the pleural space; use finger to remove any local pleural adhesions.
- **G.** Use the Kelly clamp to grasp the tip of the thoracostomy tube (36 F, Argyle, internal diameter 12 mm), and direct it into the pleural space in a posterior, superior direction for pneumothorax evacuation. Direct tube inferiorly for pleural fluid removal. Guide the tube into the pleural space until the last hole is inside the pleural space and not inside the subcutaneous tissue.
- **H.** Attach the tube to 20 cm $H_2O$ of suction. Suture the tube to the skin of the chest wall using O silk. An untied, vertical, mattress suture may be placed in order to close the skin after removal of chest tube.
- **I.** Apply Vaseline gauze, 4 x 4 gauze sponges, and elastic tape. Obtain a chest X-ray to verify correct tube placement and to evaluate re-expansion of the lung.
- **J.** Indications for Thoracotomy After Trauma
    1. >1000 mL blood from chest tube on insertion
    2. >200 mL blood/hour from chest tube thereafter
    3. Massive air leak such that lung will not re-expand, dispite properly placed and functioning chest tube.

# Tension Pneumothorax

## I. Clinical Signs

- **A.** Severe hemodynamic and respiratory compromise; contralaterally deviated trachea; decreased or absent breath sounds on the involved side.
- **B.** Hyperresonance to percussion on the affected side; jugular venous

distention, asymmetrical chest wall motion with respiration.

## II. Radiographic Findings
A. Flattening or inversion of the ipsilateral hemidiaphragm; contralateral shifting of the mediastinum.
B. Flattening of the cardiomediastinal contour, and spreading of the ribs on the ipsilateral side.
C. Loss of lung markings of ipsilateral side.

## III. Acute Management of Tension Pneumothorax
A. Place a chest tube immediately as described above. A temporary large-bore IV catheter may be inserted into the pleural space, at the level of the second intercostal space at the mid-clavicular line, until the chest tube is placed.
B. Insert 2 large-bore intravenous lines. Intubation and central venous pressure monitoring and an arterial line may also be indicated.
C. Draw blood for CBC, PT, PTT, type and cross-matching.

# Flail Chest

## I. Clinical Evaluation
A. Usually secondary to severe, blunt, chest injury with multiple rib fractures of adjacent ribs, with more than one fracture per rib. The fractured ribs allow a rib segment without bony continuity with the rest of the chest wall, to move freely during breathing.
B. Arterial blood gases should be measured if respiratory compromise is significant. If fracture of left, lower, rib cage, rule out splenic injury with CT scan.

## II. Management of Flail Chest
A. Aggressive pulmonary suctioning and close observation for any signs of respiratory insufficiency or hypoxemia.
B. Endotracheal intubation and positive-pressure ventilation is indicated for significant cases of flail chest if blood gas analysis reveals inadequate ventilation or oxygenation, or in the multiply injured, severely compromised patient.
C. Associated injuries such as pneumothorax and hemothorax should be treated with tube thoracostomy.
D. Pain control with an epidural or intercostal blockade may eliminate the need for intubation. Intubation is required if there are significant injuries with massive pulmonary contusion or poor pulmonary reserve.
E. If mechanical ventilation is required, the ventilator should be set to assist control mode to put the flail segment at rest for several days. Thereafter, a trial of low rate, intermittent, mandatory ventilation may be attempted to check for return of flail, prior to attempting extubation.

# Massive Hemothorax

### I. Clinical Evaluation
  A. Defined as >1500 mL blood lost into the thoracic cavity; most commonly secondary to penetrating injuries.
  B. Absence of breath sounds and dullness to percussion on the ipsilateral side; signs of hypovolemic shock.

### II. Management
  A. Simultaneously restore volume deficit and decompress chest cavity with a chest tube. Consult cardiothoracic surgeon as soon as possible.
  B. Place two large-bore intravenous lines or a central venous line.
  C. Insert a chest tube as described previously, except place the site of insertion at the level of the fifth or sixth intercostal space, along the midaxillary line, ipsilateral to the hemothorax. The chest tube should be inserted in a location away from the injury, and it should not be inserted through the injury site.
  D. Clean and close the penetrating wound, and cover it with Vaseline impregnated gauze to decrease the likelihood of tension pneumothorax.
  E. A thoracotomy is indicated if blood loss continues through the chest tube. (>200 mL/hr for 2-3 consecutive hours). If the site of wound penetration is medial to the nipple anteriorly or medial to the scapula posteriorly, this represents a higher probability for injury to the myocardium and the great vessels. If the wound is below the fourth intercostal space, abdominal injury is possible and must be assessed.
  F. Consider tetanus prophylaxis and empirical antibiotic coverage.

# Cardiac Tamponade

### I. Clinical Evaluation
  A. Cardiac Tamponade most commonly secondary to penetrating injuries. Cardiac Tamponade can also occur when a central line penetrates the wall of the right atrium.
  B. Cardiac Tamponade is often manifested by Beck's Triad of Venous pressure elevation, drop in the arterial pressure, muffled heart sounds.
  C. **Other Signs Include:** Signs and symptoms of hypovolemic shock; pulseless electrical activity (electromechanical dissociation); decreased voltage on ECG, enlarged cardiac silhouette on CXR.
  D. **Kussmaul's Sign:** Rise in venous pressure with inspiration. Pulsus paradoxus or elevated venous pressure may be absent when associated with hypovolemia.

### II. Management
  A. Pericardiocentesis or pericardial window is indicated if patient is unresponsive to fluid resuscitation measures for hypovolemic shock, and tamponade is suspected.
  B. All patients who have a positive pericardiocentesis (recovery of non-clotting blood) due to trauma, require open thoracotomy with inspection of the myocardium and the great vessels. Immediately consult cardiothoracic surgery.
  C. Temporize with IVF or blood on way to OR.
  D. Consider other causes of hemodynamic instability or electromechanical

dissociation that may mimic cardiac tamponade, such as tension pneumothorax, massive pulmonary embolism, or hypovolemic shock.
E. Subxiphoid pericardial window is as rapid and safer than pericardiocentesis if equipment and experienced surgical personel are available. If not, pericardiocentesis should be done.

# Pericardiocentesis

## I. Management
A. Infusion of Ringer's lactate, crystalloid, colloid, and/or blood may provide a temporizing measure.
B. Protect airway; unstable patients require intubation. If the patient can be stabilized, pericardiocentesis or a subxiphoid pericardial window should be accomplished in the operating room.
C. Place patient in supine position. Cleanse and drape peri-xiphoid area, and infiltrate lidocaine 1% with epinephrine into the skin and deep tissues (if time permits).
D. Attach a long, large bore (12-18 cm, 16-18 gauge), short bevel, cardiac needle to a 50 cc syringe with a 3-way stop cock. Attach a V-lead of the ECG to the metal of the needle with an alligator clip if time permits.
E. Advance the needle just below costal margin, immediately to the left and inferior to the xiphoid process. Apply suction to the syringe while advancing the needle, slowly, at a 45 degree angle towards the mid point of the left clavicle.
F. As the needle penetrates the pericardium, resistance will be felt, and a characteristic "popping" sensation will be noted.
G. Monitor the ECG for ST segment elevation (indicating ventricular heart muscle contact); or PR segment elevation (indicating atrial epicardial contact). After the needle comes in contact with the epicardium, withdraw the needle slightly. Ectopic ventricular beats are associated with cardiac penetration.
H. Aspirate as much blood as possible. Blood from the pericardial space usually will not clot. Blood, inadvertently, drawn from inside the ventricles or atrium usually will clot. If fluid is not obtained, withdraw and redirect the needle in a more medial direction.
I. Stabilize the needle by attaching a hemostat or Kelly clamp.
J. Consider emergency thoracotomy to determine the cause of hemopericardium if the patient develops profound hypotension (<70mm Hg), otherwise definite treatment is best achieved in the operating room.
K. If the patient does not improve, consider other problems that may resemble tamponade, such as tension pneumothorax, pulmonary embolism, or shock secondary to massive hemothorax.

# Other Life-Threatening Trauma Emergencies

## I. Cardiac Contusions
   **A.** Anythmias are the most common consequence of cardiac contusions, but pump failure can also occur.
   **B. Treatment:** The patient should receive cardiac monitoring for 48 hours and arrhythmias should be treated. If pump failure is suspected, assess cardiac function with an echocardiogram and/or Swan Ganz, and provide ionotropic support.

## II. Pulmonary Contusions
   **A.** Pulmonary contusions are the most common potentially lethal chest injuries following blunt chest trauma. Respiratory failure and hypoxemia may develop gradually over several hours. A continuing index of suspicion is required to make the diagnosis. The clinical severity of hypoxia does not correlate well with chest x-ray.
   **B.** If pulmonary compromise is mild and the patient is not multiply injured, selected patients can be managed without intubation.
   **C.** Treatment of significant contusions, especially in multiply injured patients, consists of intubation, positive pressure ventilation, and PEEP.

## III. Traumatic Aortic Transection
   **A.** Diagnosis requires a high index of suspicion in patients with an appropriate mechanism of injury.
   **B.** The chest x-ray may show a widened mediastiinum, obscured aortic knob, or left pleural cap. The diagnostic gold standard remains aortogram, although transesophageal echocardiogram and spiral CT scan are gaining acceptance.

## IV. Pelvic Fracture
   **A.** Fracture of the pelvis can produce exsanguinating hemorrhage. Diagnosis is by physical exam, plain x-ray films, and CT scan.
   **B.** Hemorrhage is difficult or impossible to control at laparotomy. Most bleeding is venous, and is best treated acutely by external fixation of the pelvis. Arterial bleeding sometimes occurs, and requires angiographic embolization.
   **C.** Pelvic fractures are often associated with abdominal injury. Diagnostic peritoneal lavage can be utilized to establish the presence of internal hemorrhage. Associated bladder or uretheral injuries are also common.

## V. Extremity Fractures:
Femur fractures, especially bilateral, can cause hemorrhage of several units of blood which can be life threatening, especially in elderly or multiply injured patients.

## VI. Traumatic Esophageal Injuries
   **A. Clinical Evaluation:** Eosphageal injuries are usually caused by penetrating chest injuries or severe blunt trauma to the abdomen, or by a nasogastric tube or endoscopy, or by repeated vomiting (Boerneave'e syndrome).
   **B.** After rupture, esophageal contents leak into the mediastinum, followed by immediate or delayed rupture into the pleural space (usually on left), with resulting empyema.
   **C.** A high index of suapicion is required, particularly in transthoracic penetrating injuries. Transmediastinal penetrating injuries mandate a workup for great vessel, tracheobronchial, and esophageal injuries.
   **D. Treatment of Esophageal Injuries**
      **1.** Surgical therapy consists of primary repair, or esophageal diversion in

# Burns

Bruce M. Achauer, M.D.

## I. Immediate Management of Burns

A. Stop the burning process by removing hot clothing, cool the wound with tepid water or saline (but avoid hypothermia), irrigate chemical burns; remove victim from electrical source.

B. Establish airway and administer oxygen, establish intravenous line.

C. **Airway maintenance.**
1. The airway takes first priority. Smoke inhalation should be suspected if fire occurred in a closed space or if there are thermal injuries to the face, nares, or upper torso. Examine nasal passages for soot, swelling or burns of the nasal vibrissae. Intubation is indicated if there is any evidence of an upper airway burn.
2. Blood gases, including carboxyhemoglobin, should be determined. If the patient has extreme air hunger or is in critical condition, endotracheal intubation is indicated.
3. Once intubated, leave endotracheal tube in place at least 72 hours. The tube must be well secured with a tie around the head. Tape will not be adequate to hold tube.

### Assessment of Percentage of Burn Area

| | |
|---|---|
| Head | 9% |
| Anterior Trunk | 1% |
| Posterior Trunk | 18% |
| Anterior Leg | 9% |
| Posterior Leg | 9% |
| Arm | 9% |
| Genitalia | 1% |

A. Burns involving more than 15% of the total body surface area in adults, or more than 10% in children, should be transferred to a burn center. Patients with other severe injuries, extremes of age or inhalation injury should also be admitted to a burn center.

B. **Fluid Resuscitation**
1. Place at least two 16 gauge IV catheters, arterial line, and consider a central line.
2. A urinary catheter should be inserted.

3. Administer crystalloid solution (Ringer's lactate) during the first 24 hours. The amount of crystalloid solution administered should be determined by blood pressure, pulse, and urinary output; formulas are useful guidelines but should not be adhered to rigidly if circumstances dictate otherwise.
4. The Parkland formula may be used as a guide to fluid requirements: First 24 hours--balanced salt solution (lactated Ringer's injection), 4 mL/kg/%burn; give half of this during the first 8 hours and the other half over the next 16 hours. Colloid 0.3-0.5 cc/% burn/kg body weight may also be given. Fluid requirements should be modified for each patient based on their perfusion.
5. Monitoring of fluid resuscitation: Fluid orders should be adjusted hourly. Urine output remains the best means of monitoring resuscitation. 0.5 mL/kg/hour is the acceptable minimal output in adults; 1 mL/kg/hour in children. Peripheral perfusion and sensorium should also be followed.
6. Children may require more free water than older patients; this can be monitored by frequent determinations of serum osmolality or serum sodium. Urine specific gravity can also be used to assess the amount of free water needed.

## I. Assessment of Burns

**A. First Degree Burn.** Involves epidermis only (sunburn); blanching erythema; very painful; not included in the estimation of extent of burn injury.

**B. Second Degree Burn.** Destruction of epidermis with extension into underlying dermis.

**C. Third Degree Burn.** Involves destruction of epidermis and dermis, with extension into subcutaneous tissue; painless.

**D. Fourth Degree Burn.** Extend into subcutaneous tissue, muscle, fascia, or bone.

## II. Medications

**A. Pain Control.** Initially IV morphine 0.1 mg/kg; or meperidine 1-2 mg/kg should be given to relieve all pain. Give pain medications before severe pain occurs, on an hourly basis (not "as needed").

**B.** Diazepam 5-10 mg IV doses may be given after circulation has stabilized.

**C.** Intravenous $H_2$ blockers should be routinely administered.

**D. Antibiotics.** Not given prophylactically. If a patient becomes febrile, hypotensive, anuric, hypothermic, or deteriorates despite adequate fluids, the most likely diagnosis is sepsis. After taking appropriate cultures, broad spectrum antibiotics should be given.

**E.** Tetanus toxoid (0.5 cc) should be administered to all patients. If the wound is >50% of the body surface area, 250 units of tetanus immune globulin (human) should also be administered.

## III. Burn Wound Management

**A.** Initial examination and debridement can occur during fluid resuscitation.

**B.** The burn should be initially thoroughly cleaned with sterile saline and antibacterial solution (normal saline: iodoform in a 2:1 dilation). Avoid vigorous scrubbing. Use sterile scissors to remove the charred epithelium, surface debris; leave unbroken blisters intact. Rinse with copious amounts of normal saline.

**C.** After cleaning of burns, they should be dressed with occlusive dressings combined with antibacterial cream (usually silver sulfadiazine). The ointment or cream may be applied to the patient or to the gauze. The

cream should then be covered with elastic gauze netting.
- **D.** Silver sulfadiazine may cause transitory leukopenia, due to margination of white cells. This leukopenia is benign and does not necessitate discontinuing the drug.
- **E.** Burn areas that are full thickness or deep partial thickness should be excised and grafted during the first few post-burn days.
- **F.** Burns that will heal in 14-21 days are best treated nonsurgically.
- **G.** Patients should be bathed daily at which time the dressings or cream are washed off. Debridement of all loose tissues is performed during the bath.
- **H. Extremity Burns**
    1. Circumferential burns and subsequent edema may impair circulation. Impaired circulation must be relieved by escharotomy.
    2. Prior to escharotomy, tissue pressure should be monitored clinically, or by tissue pressure measurements until pressure measurements have been less than 40 mmHg for more than 72 hours.
    3. Hand burns should be splinted in the anti-claw position and physical therapy should be initiated immediately.

**References:** See page 106.

# *Pulmonology*

Charles F. Chandler, M.D.

## Airway Management and Intubation

**Orotracheal Intubation:**
**ETT Size** (interior diameter):
>Women 7.0-9.0 mm
>Men    8.0-10.0 mm.

1. **Prepare functioning suction** apparatus. Have bag and mask apparatus set-up with 100% oxygen; and ensure that patient can be adequately bagged and suction apparatus is available.
2. **If sedation and/or paralysis is required,** consider rapid sequence induction as follows:
   - Fentanyl (Sublimaze) 50 mcg increments IV (1 mcg/kg) **with:**
   - Midazolam hydrochloride (Versed) 1 mg IV q2-3 min, max 0.1-0.15 mg/kg **followed by:**
   - Succinylcholine (Anectine) 0.6-1.0 mg/kg, at appropriate intervals.

   **Note:** These drugs may cause vomiting; therefore, cricoid cartilage pressure should be applied during intubation (Sellick maneuver).
3. **Position the patient's head** in "sniffing" position with head flexed at neck and extended. If necessary elevate head with a small pillow.
4. **Ventilate patient** with bag mask apparatus and hyperoxygenate with 100% oxygen.
5. **Hold Endoscope handle** with left hand, and use right hand to open patient's mouth. Insert blade along the right side of mouth to the base of tongue, and push the tongue to the left. If using curved blade, advance to the vallecula (superior to epiglottis), and lift anteriorly, being careful not to exert pressure on the teeth. If using a straight blade, place beneath the epiglottis and lift anteriorly.
6. **Place endotracheal tube (ETT)** into right corner of mouth and pass it through the vocal cords; stop just after the cuff disappears behind vocal cords. If unsuccessful after 30 seconds, stop and resume bag and mask ventilation before reattempting. If necessary, use stilette to maintain the shape of the ETT (a hockey stick shape may be helpful); remove stilette after intubation. Application of lubricant jelly at endotracheal tube balloon facilitates passage through the vocal cords.
7. **Inflate cuff with syringe** keeping cuff pressure $\leq 20$ cm $H_2O$ and attach the tube to an Ambu bag or ventilator. Confirm bilateral, equal expansion of the chest and equal bilateral breath sounds. Auscultate abdomen to confirm that the ETT is not in the esophagus. If there is any question about proper ETT location, repeat laryngoscopy with tube in place to be sure it is endotracheal; remove tube immediately if there is any doubt about proper location. Secure the tube with tape and note centimeter mark at the mouth. Suction the oropharynx and trachea.
8. **Confirm proper tube placement with a chest X-ray** (tip of ETT should be between the carina and thoracic inlet, or level with the top of the aortic

notch).

**Nasotracheal Intubation:**
Nasotracheal intubation is the preferred method if prolonged intubation is anticipated (increased patient comfort). Intubation will be facilitated if patient is awake and spontaneously breathing. There is an increased incidence of sinusitis with nasotracheal intubation.

1. **Spray nasal passage with a vasoconstrictor** such as cocaine 4% or phenylephrine 0.25% (Neo-Synephrine) may be used. If sedation is required before nasotracheal intubation, administer fentanyl (Sublimaze) 1 mcg/kg with midazolam hydrochloride (Versed) 0.05-0.1 mg/kg.
   Lubricate nasal airway with lidocaine ointment.
   **Tube Size:**
   Women   7.0 mm tube
   Men   8.0, 9.0 mm tube
2. **Place the nasotracheal tube into the nasal passage** and guide it into nasopharynx along a U-shaped path. Monitor breath sounds by listening and feeling the end of tube. As the tube enters the oropharynx, gradually guide the tube downward. If the breath sounds stop, withdraw the tube 1-2 cm until breath sounds are heard again. Reposition the tube, and, if necessary, extend the head and advance. If difficulty is encountered, perform direct laryngoscopy and insert tube under direct visualization, or use Magill forceps.
3. **Successful intubation** occurs when the tube passes through the cords; a cough may occur and breath sounds will reach maximum intensity if the tube is correctly positioned. Confirm correct placement by checking for bilateral breath sounds and expansion of chest.
4. **Confirm proper tube placement** with chest x-ray.

# Ventilator Management

I. **Indications for Ventilatory Support:** Respirations >35, vital capacity <15 mL/kg, negative inspiratory force $\leq$-25, pO2 <60 on 50% $O_2$, pH <7.2, $pCO_2$ $\geq$55, severe, progressive, symptomatic hypercapnia and/or hypoxia, severe metabolic acidosis.

II. **Initiation of Ventilator Support**
   A. **Intubation**
      1. Prepare suction apparatus, laryngoscope, endotracheal tube ($\geq$ No. 8 if possible); clear airway and place oral airway, hyperventilate with bag and mask attached to high flow oxygen.
      2. Midazolam (Versed) 1-2 mg IV boluses until sedated.
      3. Intubate, inflate cuff, ventilate with bag, auscultate chest, and suction trachea.
   B. **Initial Orders:** $FiO_2$ = 100%, PEEP = 3-5 cm $H_2O$, assist control 8-14 breaths/min, tidal volume = 800 mL (10-15 mL/kg ideal body weight), set rate so that minute ventilation (VE) is approximately 10 L/min. Alternatively, use intermittent mandatory ventilation mode with tidal volume and rate to achieve near-total ventilatory support. Consider pressure support in addition to IMV at 5-15 cm $H_2O$.
   C. ABG should be obtained in 30 min, CXR for tube placement, measure

cuff pressure q8h (maintain ≤20 mm Hg), pulse oximeter, arterial line, and/or monitor end tidal $CO_2$. Maintain oxygen saturation >90-95%.

## D. Ventilator Management

1. **Decreased Minute Ventilation:** Evaluate patient and rule out complications (endotracheal tube malposition, cuff leak, excessive secretions, bronchospasms, pneumothorax, worsening pulmonary disease, sedative drugs, pulmonary infection). Readjust ventilator rate to maintain mechanically assisted minute ventilation of 10 L/min. If peak airway pressure (AWP) is >45 cm $H_2O$, decrease tidal volume to 7-8 mL/kg (with increase in rate if necessary), or decrease ventilator flow rate.

2. **Arterial Saturation ≥94% and $pO_2$ >100**, reduce $FIO_2$ (each 1% decrease in $FIO_2$ reduces $pO_2$ by 7 mm Hg); once $FIO_2$ is <60%, PEEP may be reduced by increments of 2 cm $H_2O$ until PEEP = 3-5 cm $H_2O$. Maintain $O_2$ saturation of ≥90% ($pO_2$ >60).

3. **Arterial saturation <90% and pO2 <60,** increase $FIO_2$ up to 60-100%, then consider increasing PEEP by increments of 3-5 cm $H_2O$ (PEEP >10 requires a PA catheter). Add additional PEEP until oxygenation is adequate with an $FIO_2$ of <60%.

4. **Excessively Low pH,** (pH <7.33 because of respiratory acidosis/hypercapnia): Increase rate and/or tidal volume. Keep peak airway pressure <40-50 cm $H_2O$ if possible.

5. **Excessively High pH** (>7.48 because of respiratory alkalosis/hypocapnia): Reduce rate and/or tidal volume to lessen hyperventilation. If patient is breathing rapidly above ventilator rate, sedate patient.

6. **Patient "Fighting" Ventilator:** Consider IMV or SIMV mode, or add sedation with or without paralysis (exclude complications or other causes of agitation). Paralytic agents should not be used without concurrent amnesia and/or sedation.

7. **Sedation:**
   a. Diazepam (Valium) 2-5 mg slow IV q2h prn agitation **OR**
   b. Lorazepam (Ativan) 1-2 mg IV q1-2h prn sedation **OR**
   c. Midazolam (Versed) 0.5-1 mg IV boluses until sedated.
   d. Morphine Sulfate 2-5 mg IV q5min, max dose 20-30 mg OR 0.03-0.05 mg/kg/h IV infusion (50-100 mg in 500 mL D5W) titrated **OR**
   e. Propofol (Diprivan): 50 mcg/kg bolus over 5 min, then 5-50 mcg/kg/min.

8. **Paralysis (with simultaneous sedation and/or amnesia):**
   a. Succinylcholine (Anectine) 0.6-1.0 mg/kg; short acting, T1/2 3.5 min **OR**
   b. Vecuronium (Norcuron) 0.1 mg/kg IV, then 0.06 mc/kg/h IV infusion or q1h prn; intermediate acting, T1/2 60 min; no hemodynamic or cardiac depressive effects **OR**
   c. Pancuronium (Pavulon) 0.08 mg/kg IV, then 0.05 mg/kg/h infusion or q1h IV prn; long acting, T1/2 75 min; may cause tachycardia and/or hypertension **OR**
   d. Atracurium (Tracrium) 0.5 mg/kg IV, then 0.3-0.6 mg/kg/h infusion; short acting, T1/2 20 min; because of histamine releasing properties, may cause bronchospasm and/or hypotension.
   e. Monitor level of paralysis with a peripheral nerve stimulator.

Adjust neuromuscular blocker dosage to achieve a "train-of-four" (TOF) of 90-95%; if patient on inverse ratio ventilation is used, maintain TOF at 100%.
9. **Loss of Tidal Volume:** If a difference between the tidal volume setting and the delivered volume occurs, check for a leak in the ventilator or inspiratory line. Check for a poor seal between the endotracheal tube cuff or malposition of the cuff in the subglottic area. If a chest tube is present, check for air leak.
10. **Daily weaning parameters** should be obtained when weaning is being considered.

# Epistaxis

Almost all persons have experienced a nosebleed at some time, and most nosebleeds resolve without requiring medical attention. Prolonged epistaxis, however, can be life-threatening, especially the elderly or debilitated.

I. **Pathophysiology**
   A. **Anterior epistaxis**, in the anterior two thirds of the nose, is visible on the septum, and is the most common type of epistaxis. Anterior bleeding can often be resolved by pinching the cartilaginous part of the nose.
   B. **Posterior epistaxis** from the posterior third of the nose accounts for 10% of nosebleeds. Bleeding is profuse because of the larger vessels in that location. Posterior epistaxis usually occurs in older patients, who have fragile vessels because of hypertension, atherosclerosis, coagulopathies, or weakened tissue. Posterior bleeds require aggressive treatment and hospitalization.
   C. The anterior portion of the septum has a rich vascular supply, known as Kiesselbach's plexus, or Little's area, and most epistaxis originates in this region. Posterior hemorrhages originate from larger vessels near the sphenopalatine artery, behind the middle turbinate.

II. **Causes of Epistaxis**
   A. **Trauma.** Nose picking, nose blowing, or sneezing can tear or abrade the mucosa and cause bleeding. Other forms of trauma include nasal fracture and nasogastric and nasotracheal intubation.
   B. **Desiccation.** Cold, dry air, and dry heat contribute to an increased incidence of epistaxis during the winter.
   C. **Other causes of nasal drying** include dehydration (eg, from poorly controlled diabetes mellitus), nasal sprays (eg, corticosteroids and cromolyn), and nasal oxygen therapy.
   D. **Irritation.** Upper respiratory infections, sinusitis, allergies, topical decongestants, and cocaine sniffing cause increased vulnerability to bleeding.
   E. **Hereditary Hemorrhagic Telangiectasia.** This autosomal dominant condition weakens the capillaries and causes bleeding.
   F. **Nasal Septal Disease.** Less common causes of anterior epistaxis include Wegener's granulomatosis, mid-line destructive disease, tuberculosis, and syphilis.
   G. **Systemic Disease.** Epistaxis will be exacerbated by coagulopathy, blood dyscrasia, thrombocytopenia, or anticoagulant medication (NSAIDs, warfarin), hepatic cirrhosis, and renal failure.

## Epistaxis

- **H. Hypertension** complicates active bleeding by promoting rigid arteries, and arteriosclerosis weakens vessels and inhibits vasoconstriction. These risk factors contribute to the posterior epistaxis most often seen in elderly patients.
- **I. Tumors.** Juvenile nasopharyngeal angiofibroma, a benign, tumor, can cause profuse, life-threatening posterior epistaxis. Inverted papilloma less commonly presents with bleeding. Malignant neoplasms such as squamous cell carcinoma, adenocarcinoma, melanoma, esthesioneuroblastoma, and lymphoma can cause epistaxis.
- **J. Foreign Bodies.** A foreign body should be considered when a child has unilateral nasal obstruction, new-onset snoring, halitosis, or epistaxis.

### III. Clinical Evaluation of Epistaxis

- **A.** Hemodynamic evaluation for tachycardia, hypotension, light-headedness should be completed immediately. Hypovolemic patients should be resuscitated with fluids and packed red blood cells.
- **B.** After stabilization, the site, cause, and amount of bleeding is determined. Most patients require no immediate resuscitation. Posterior epistaxis in an elderly and debilitated patient can be life-threatening because of aspiration, hypoxia, exsanguination, or myocardial infarction.
- **C. Determine the side on which the bleeding occurred:** Unilateral nose bleeding suggests anterior epistaxis in Kiesselbach's plexus. Bilateral bleeding suggests posterior epistaxis caused by overflow around the posterior septum.
- **D. Determine whether epistaxis is anterior or posterior:** When the patient is upright, blood drains primarily from the anterior part of the nose in anterior bleeding, or it drains from the nasopharynx in posterior bleeding.
- **E. Assess the duration** of the nosebleed and any inciting incident (eg, trauma). Swallowed blood from epistaxis may cause melena.
- **F. Medical History:** Hypertension, bleeding disorders, diabetes, alcoholism, liver disease, pulmonary disease, cardiac disease, arteriosclerosis should be assessed.
- **G. Medications** including aspirin or aspirin-containing products, other NSAIDs, warfarin, nasal sprays, and oxygen via nasal cannula should be sought.
- **H. Blood Tests**
    1. Hematologic tests include CBC, platelet counts, prothrombin time, and partial thromboplastin time, and blood for type and cross in case a transfusion is needed.
    2. The hematocrit does not immediately drop in acute hemorrhage because time is required for fluid dilution of blood.

### IV. Location of the Site of Bleeding

- **A. Sedation:** When sedation is required, midazolam (Versed), 1-2 mg IV in adults and 0.035-0.2 mg/kg IV in children is recommended; overmedication may threaten the cough reflex that protects the airway.
- **B. Drape the patient**, and furnish a spit basin. Keep the patient sitting upright or leaning forward. Wear a gown, gloves, mask, and protective eyewear because patients may inadvertently cough blood.
- **C. A nasal speculum** and a suction apparatus with a #10 Frazier tip are used to aspirate blood from the nose and oropharynx.
- **D. Anesthesia and Vasoconstriction:** A cotton-tipped applicator or cotton pledget is used to apply a topical anesthetic (eg, 1% tetracaine or 4%

# Epistaxis

lidocaine) and a topical vasoconstrictor (eg, 1% ephedrine, 1% phenylephrine, or 0.05% oxymetazoline) to the entire nasal mucosa, especially to the septum, inferior turbinate, posterior middle turbinate, and superior mucosa. These agents take effect in 5 to 10 minutes. If a bleeding site is observed, press the vasoconstrictor applicator directly to that site.

### E. Visualization of Bleeding Site
1. Use the nasal speculum to facilitate exposure, taking care to minimize further mucosal injury. Apply suction to remove blood and clots.
2. Localize active bleeding. Kiesselbach's plexus and the inferior turbinate are the most frequent sites of bleeding.
3. If blood is spilling from the superior aspect of the nose, the ethmoidal arteries may be involved, usually following facial trauma.
4. Posterior bleeding may be located by applying suction; when the suction tip is at the site of bleeding, blood will no longer well up.

## V. Management of Hemorrhage

### A. 
Anterior septal hemorrhage can sometimes be stopped by nose pinching alone. Have the patient sit upright to decrease venous pressure. If bleeding continues, application of the topical anesthetic and vasoconstrictor may stop it.

### B. Cauterization
1. Bleeding sites that can be visualized should be cauterized with silver nitrate sticks; they work best in a dry field accomplished by vasoconstriction and suction.
2. Press or roll the silver nitrate over the bleeding site for several seconds, allowing a gray eschar to form.
3. The septum should not be cauterized bilaterally at the same level because it may cause cartilaginous necrosis and septal perforation.

### C. Hemostatic Agents
1. Application of a hemostatic material (eg, microfibrillar collagen or oxidized regenerated cellulose) to the bleeding site may be useful. These products do not require removal because they dissolve in the nose after several days. The patient should lubricate the nose regularly with saline nasal spray and to use bacitracin ointment tid.

### D. Packing: 
Gauze packing or a sponge pack applied to the anterior portion of the nose are used as a tamponade for uncontrolled bleeding sites. These packs stay in place for 5 days.

### E. Anterior Nasal Pack
1. The pack consists of 72 inches of half-inch gauze impregnated with antibiotic ointment (eg, bacitracin). Topical anesthesia is necessary.
2. Use the nasal speculum to open the vestibule vertically. With the bayonet forceps, grasp the gauze approximately 10 cm from the end; place a layer along the floor of the nose all the way back to the nasopharynx. The loose end should protrude from the nose. Reposition the speculum on top of the first layer and apply another layer. Fill the entire nose with gauze, and apply a nasal drip pad.
3. **An Oral Broad-spectrum Antibiotic**, such as cephalexin (Keflex), 500 mg orally every 6 hours, is given while the pack is in place to prevent secondary sinusitis or toxic shock syndrome.
4. The pack may obstruct the nasolacrimal duct, causing tearing or retrograde bleeding from the lacrimal puncture at the medial canthus.

5. The pack is removed after 5 days.
- F. **Sponge Pack**
    1. A newer variation of the anterior pack consists of a dry, compressed sponge. The sponge is lubricated with an antibiotic ointment, then placed into the nasal cavity. Once moistened with blood or saline, the sponge expands, filling the nasal cavity and exerting gentle pressure on the bleeding site.
    2. Moisten the pack before removal after 5 days.
- G. **Posterior Pack**
    1. Posterior bleeding requires a posterior a pack, and the patient should be admitted to the hospital.
    2. The posterior pack requires a sphenopalatine block and topical anesthetic.
    3. The posterior pack is made by sewing together two tonsil tampons with 0-silk, leaving two 8-inch tails, and lubricating the tampons with antibiotic ointment.
    4. Pass the red rubber catheter through the involved nostril to the oropharynx and out the mouth. Attach the free ends of the silk sutures to the oral end of the catheter, and pull the catheter back out of the nose, pulling the tampons into the nasopharynx while guiding them with your fingers, and lodge them snugly into the involved choana. Be sure the uvula is free.
    5. Trim the loose cotton tampon tails at the level of the uvula to facilitate pack removal.
    6. Have an assistant hold the packs firmly in place by applying traction to the silk tails as they exit the nostril.
    7. Place a tight anterior gauze pack, and tie the tails around one or two dental rolls to stabilize the tampons.
    8. The patient is admitted to the hospital for airway observation, administration of humidified air or oxygen, mild sedation, and antibiotics. Elevate the head of the bed at least 30 degrees. Cold foods and liquids are given, and ambulation is allowed after 12-24 hours.
    9. The pack is removed after 5 days.
- H. **Balloon Pack**
    1. A popular alternative to the tampon posterior pack is a 14-French, 30-mL balloon Foley catheter.
    2. Use the same anesthetic as for the tampon posterior pack, and cover the balloon with antibiotic ointment, and insert it through the nostril until the tip can be seen in the nasopharynx.
    3. Inflate the balloon with 10 to 12 mL of saline or water, and lodge it in the choana using anterior traction.
    4. Place an anterior pack around the catheter back to the balloon.
    5. Secure the Foley catheter under traction, using an umbilical clamp, protecting the ala with thick gauze pads.
    6. The advantages of this procedure include ease of placement, relative patient comfort, and the ability to test adequate hemostasis by deflating the balloon.
- VI. **Management of Refractory Epistaxis**: Patients who continue to bleed after a snug posterior pack is in place, may require endoscopic cautery, radiographic embolization or surgical ligation of the arterial supply to the bleeding area.

**48 Epistaxis**

# Disorders of the Alimentary Tract

John Craig Collins, M.D.
Russell A. Williams, M.D.
I. James Sarfeh, M.D.

## Acute Abdomen

I. **Clinical Evaluation**
   A. Duration, acuity, and progression of pain; exact location of maximal pain at onset and at present; diffuse or localized. Time course of pain (constant, intermittent, decreasing, increasing).
   B. Character at onset and at present (crampy, sharp, dull); constant or intermittent; radiation (to shoulder, mid-back, groin); sudden or gradual onset.
   C. Effect of eating, vomiting, defecation, passing of gas, urination, inspiration, movement, position, last bowel movement, menstrual period. Similar episodes in past.
   D. **Associated Symptoms:** Fever, chills, nausea, vomiting (bilious, feculent, food, blood, coffee grounds); vomiting before or after onset of pain; chest pain; constipation, change in bowel habits or stool caliber; obstipation (inability to pass gas); diarrhea, hematochezia (rectal bleeding), melena (black stools), dysuria, anorexia, weight loss, early satiety.
   E. **Past Medical History:** Abdominal surgery (appendectomy, cholecystectomy), hernias, gallstones; coronary disease, kidney stones; alcohol intake, dyspepsia. Past treatment or testing, endoscopies, x-rays.
   F. **Aggravating or Relieving Factors:** Fatty food intolerance, medications, aspirin, NSAID's. Use of narcotics, anticholinergics, laxatives, antacids.

II. **Physical Exam**
   A. **General:** Degree of distress; severity of pain; nutritional status; activity (moving to relieve pain or lying still to prevent pain).
   B. **Vital Signs:** T (fever), P (tachycardia), BP (hypotension), R (tachypnea).
   C. **HEENT:** Oral signs of dehydration (lack of oral moisture, fissured tongue); signs of upper respiratory infection.
   D. **Chest:** Rhonchi or rales may indicate lower lobe pneumonia that may cause upper abdominal pain.
   E. **Abdomen:**
      1. **Inspection:** Scars, evidence of trauma, visible peristalsis (small bowel obstruction), distention.
      2. **Auscultation:** Absent bowel sounds (paralytic ileus or late obstruction), high-pitched rushes (obstruction), bruits (ischemic colitis).
      3. **Palpation:** Begin palpation in quadrant diagonally opposite to point of maximal pain with patient's legs relaxed and slightly flexed. Bimanual palpation of flank may reveal renal disease or retrocecal appendicitis. Rebound tenderness, hepatomegaly, splenomegaly, masses; hernias (incisional, inguinal, femoral). Pulsating masses; costovertebral angle tenderness. Shifting dullness (ascites). Cutaneous hyperesthesia (pain with light touch, indicates parietal peritoneal inflation of appendicitis).

## 50 Acute Abdomen

4. **Specific Abdominal Signs**
   a. **Murphy's sign:** Inspiratory arrest with right upper quadrant palpation, cholecystitis.
   b. **Charcot's Triad:** Right upper quadrant pain, jaundice, fever; gallstones.
   c. **Courvoisier's sign:** Palpable, nontender gallbladder with jaundice, pancreatic malignancy.
   d. **McBurney's Point Tenderness:** Located two thirds of the way between umbilicus and anterior superior iliac spine, appendicitis.
   e. **Iliopsoas Sign:** Elevation of legs against examiner's hand causes pain, retrocecal appendicitis.
   f. **Obturator Sign:** Flexion of right thigh and external rotation of thigh causes pain in pelvic appendicitis.
   g. **Rovsing's Sign:** Manual pressure and release at left lower quadrant colon causes referred pain at McBurney's point (referred rebound tenderness from appendicitis).
   h. **Cullen's Sign:** Bluish periumbilical discoloration, peritoneal hemorrhage.
5. **Percussion:** Loss of liver dullness indicates perforated viscus and free air in peritoneum; liver and spleen span by percussion.

F. **Rectal:** Masses, tenderness, feces; gross or occult blood. Bimanual palpation of the lower abdomen may elicit concealed tenderness or mass.
G. **Genital/Pelvic Examination:** Adnexal tenderness, cervical discharge, uterine size, masses, cervical motion tenderness.
H. **Extremities:** Femoral pulses, popliteal pulses (absent pulses may indicate ischemic colitis).
I. **Skin:** Jaundice, dependent purpura (mesenteric infarction), petechia (gonococcemia).
J. **Stigmata of Liver Disease:** Spider angiomata, periumbilical collateral veins (Caput medusae), gynecomastia, ascites, hepatosplenomegaly, testicular atrophy.

III. **Laboratory Evaluation of the Acute Abdomen**
   A. CBC, electrolytes, liver function tests, amylase, lipase, UA. Serum beta-HCG, ECG; chest x-ray: free air under diaphragm.
   B. **Acute Abdomen Series:** Includes upright PA chest, plain abdominal film ("flat plate"), upright film and left lateral decubitus; check for flank stripe, air fluid levels, mass effect, calcifications, fecaliths, absent bowel gas in RLQ (appendicitis), aortic aneurysm. Free air, widening of spaces between loops of bowel (thickening of bowel wall), and "ground glass" appearance of ascites may be seen.

IV. **Differential Diagnosis**
   A. **Generalized Pain:** Generalized peritonitis, intestinal infarction, obstruction, diabetic ketoacidosis, sickle crisis, acute porphyria, penetrating posterior duodenal ulcer, psychogenic.
   B. **Epigastrium:** Gastritis, peptic ulcer, esophagitis, gastroenteritis, pancreatitis, perforated viscus, intestinal obstruction, myocardial infarction, aortic aneurysm, ileus.
   C. **Right Upper Quadrant:** Biliary colic, cholecystitis, cholangitis, hepatitis, gastritis, pancreatitis, pneumonia, peptic ulcer, gastroesophageal reflux disease, retrocecal appendicitis, hepatic metastases, gonococcal perihepatitis (Fitz-Hugh-Curtis syndrome).
   D. **Left Upper Quadrant:** Peptic ulcer, gastritis, esophagitis, gastroesop-

hageal reflux, pancreatitis, pericarditis, myocardial ischemia, pneumonia, splenic rupture, pulmonary embolus.
- E. **Left Lower Quadrant:** Diverticulitis, intestinal obstruction, colitis, strangulated hernia, inflammatory bowel disease, pyelonephritis, nephrolithiasis, mesenteric lymphadenitis, mesenteric ischemia or thrombosis, aortic aneurysm rupture, volvulus, intussusception, salpingitis, ovarian cyst, ectopic, testicular torsion, psychogenic.
- F. **Right Lower Quadrant:** Appendicitis, diverticulitis, salpingitis, renal calculus, intussusception, ruptured ectopic pregnancy, hemorrhage or rupture of ovarian cyst, perforated cecal diverticulum, regional enteritis.
- G. **Hypogastric/Pelvic:** Cystitis, salpingitis, ectopic, endometriosis, endometritis appendicitis, diverticulitis, ovarian cyst torsion; distended bladder, hernia, nephrolithiasis, prostatitis, carcinoma.

# Management of the Acute Abdomen

## I. Acute Management
- A. **Evaluation** should be timely with a decision made on operation, or non-operation and observation. Admit for repeat examination even if the need for operation remains uncertain.
- B. **Analgesics and antibiotics** should be considered only after a presumptive diagnosis has been made. Narcotics and sedatives should be withheld until a diagnosis has been determined.
- C. **Patient should be NPO** until a definite diagnosis is determined and treatment is initiated.
- D. **IV fluids:** Maintenance fluids plus expected fluid losses. Replace prior loss if vomiting or dehydration. Nasogastric intubation and suction should be initiated if the patient is vomiting, bleeding, or has signs of intestinal obstruction.
- E. **Vital signs** q1hour. Place Foley catheter and monitor urine output.
- F. **Serial abdominal examinations** should be performed until definitive diagnosis has been made or the patient improves. Draw serial CBC q4-6 hours. If necessary, give maintenance medications by IV, IM, or by suppository.
- G. The patient should be considered to have appendicitis or other serious abdominal pathology until determined otherwise.

## II. Laboratory Testing
- A. CBC with differential, urinalysis, electrolytes, abdominal and chest x-rays. Culture of cervical discharge.
- B. Ultrasound of right upper quadrant (and upper abdomen if gallstones, common bile duct obstruction, or pancreatitis suspected). Ultrasound of lower abdomen and pelvis if symptoms of diverticulitis, pelvic inflammatory disease, appendicitis.
- C. Low pressure water soluble contrast enema or CT with contrast per rectum if suspect diverticulitis.
- D. Intravenous pyelogram (IVP) if gallstones suspected.

# Appendicitis

I. **Clinical Evaluation**
   A. **History:** Abdominal pain beginning in the epigastrium or mid abdomen then migrating to the right lower quadrant within 6 hours. Alteration in bowel function (diarrhea or constipation). Anorexia, nausea; vomiting after the onset of pain. Perforation may cause generalized peritonitis that is manifest by pain that changes from localized to diffuse.
   B. **Physical**
      1. Elevated temperature; tenderness at McBurney's point (2/3 of the way between the umbilicus and anterior superior iliac spine), decreased bowel sounds.
      2. Rebound tenderness, rigidity. Palpation of the left lower quadrant often causes referred pain to the right lower quadrant (Rovsing's sign). A mass may indicate an abscess.
      3. Iliopsoas sign (elevation and flexion-extension of right leg elicits back pain).
      4. Obturator sign (flexion of knee and rotation of leg medially causes worsening of pain, pelvic appendix).
      5. Rectal or pelvic exam elicits pain on right side; cutaneous hyperesthesia (hypersensitivity to touch in right lower quadrant).

II. **Laboratory Evaluation**
   A. WBC count (leukocytosis and left shift). Urinalysis may reveal protein, WBC's or RBC's.
   B. Upright abdominal x-ray: Absent bowel gas in the right lower quadrant with normal gas pattern in the remainder of the abdomen. Loss of the right flank stripe; a fecalith may sometimes be visible.
   C. Ultrasonography may reveal swollen appendix.
   D. Laparoscopy may be indicated if a gynecologic diagnoses is suspected.

III. **Differential Diagnosis:** Appendicitis, PID, intestinal obstruction, strangulated hernia, inflammatory bowel disease, gastroenteritis, pyelonephritis, mesenteric adenitis, mesenteric ischemia or thrombosis; nephrolithiasis, volvulus, intussusception, sickle crisis, ovarian cyst, ectopic, salpingitis, carcinoma, ketoacidosis, zoster neuritis, spinal arthritis, testicular torsion, psychogenic.

IV. **Treatment**
   A. If a clinical suspicion of appendicitis exist, then early appendectomy via right lower quadrant incision should be performed.
   B. A diagnosis should be determined within 24 hours of admission, and a decision should be made to operate or to provide conservative therapy.
   C. If a periappendiceal phlegmon is present then selected patients may be treated conservatively with broad spectrum IV antibiotics, and no oral intake. Antibiotics should cover gram negative and anaerobic organisms. Interval appendectomy can be done in 6 weeks.
   D. For an appendiceal abscess, give IV antibiotics, drain abscess via RLQ incision and remove appendix.
   E. Antibiotic (Cefoxitin, Cefotan, Timentin, or Zosyn) is given IV until resolution of ileus, absence of tenderness, and afebrile for 48 hours; usually within 5 days.

# Appendectomy Surgical Technique

1. After induction of anesthesia, place an incision over any obvious appendiceal mass if palpable. If no mass is present, make a transverse skin incision over McBurney's point, located two thirds of the way between the umbilicus and anterior superior iliac spine.
2. Incise the subcutaneous tissues in the line of the transverse incision, and incise the external oblique aponeurosis in the direction of its muscle fibers. Spread the muscle with a Peon hemostat. Incise the internal oblique fascia and spread the incision in the direction of its fibers. Sharply incise the transversus abdominis muscle, transversalis fascia, and peritoneum. Note the presence and nature of peritoneal fluid, and send purulent fluid for Gram's stain and aerobic and anaerobic culture.
3. Identify the base of the cecum by the converging taeniae coli, and raise the cecum, exposing the base of the appendix. Hook an index finger around the appendix, and gently break down any adhesions to adjacent tissues. Use gauze packing to isolate the inflamed appendix, and stabilize the appendix with a Babcock forceps.
4. Divide the mesoappendix between clamps, then firmly ligate below the clamps with 000 silk or polyglycolic acid sutures. Apply an encircling purse-string suture of 000 silk at the end of the cecum about 0.8 cm from the base of the appendix. Place a hemostat at the proximal base of the appendix, and crush the appendix. Remove the hemostat and reapply it distal to the crush, on the appendix. Use an 0 chromic catgut suture to ligate the crushed area below the hemostat.
5. Transect the appendix against the clamp. Invert the stump into the cecum with the purse string, and tie the purse-string suture, burying the stump. Irrigate the peritoneum with normal saline, and examine the mesoappendix and abdominal wall for hemostasis, then close the peritoneum with continuous 000 catgut suture.
6. Close the internal oblique and transversus abdominis with interrupted O chromic catgut. Close the external oblique as a separate layer. Close the skin and subcutaneous tissues.
7. Drains should be placed if perforation has occurred and a well-defined residual abscess cavity is present. Use a soft rubber Penrose drain and bring out through a separate stab incision in the lateral abdominal wall, located as dependently as possible.

## F. Intravenous Antibiotics

1. Antibiotic prophylaxis should include coverage for bowel flora, including aerobes and anaerobes.
2. Recommended prophylaxis: Cefoxitin (Mefoxin) or cefotetan (Cefotan) or piperacillin/tazobactam (Zosyn) should be given prophylactically before the operation and discontinued after one or two doses postoperatively unless the appendix has perforated.
3. If perforation is found, IV antibiotics should be continued for approximately 5-10 days. Check culture on third postoperative day and change antimicrobials if a resistant organism is present.

# Abdominal Hernias

## I. Classification of Hernias
   A. A hernia is an abnormal opening in the abdominal wall, with or without protrusion of an intra-abdominal structure. The most common groin hernia in either males or female is the indirect inguinal hernia. Femoral hernias are more common in females than in males.
   B. **Incarceration:** A hernia that can not be reduced; may be acute or chronic; painful or asymptomatic.
   C. **Strangulated Hernia:** An incarcerated hernia with compromised blood supply.
   D. **Sliding Hernia:** A hernia in which a portion of the hernia wall consists of either cecum or sigmoid.
   E. **Richter's Hernia:** Only a "knuckle" of bowel enters the hernia sac, and only one wall of the bowel is within the sac. Bowel incarceration can occur without bowel obstruction.

## II. Anatomy of the Inguinal Area
   A. **Layers of Abdominal Wall:** Skin, subcutaneous fat, Scarpa's fascia, external oblique, internal oblique, transversus abdominous, transversalis fascia, peritoneum.
   B. **Hesselbach's Triangle:** A triangle formed by the lateral edge of rectus sheath, the inferior epigastric vessels, and the inguinal ligament (direct hernias occur here).
   C. **Inguinal Ligament:** Ligament running from anterior superior iliac spine to the pubic tubercle.
   D. **Lacunar Ligament:** Reflection of inguinal ligament from the pubic tubercle onto the iliopectinal line of the pubic ramus.
   E. **Cooper's Ligament:** Strong, fibrous band located on the iliopectinal line of superior public ramus (used for McVay repair).
   F. **External Inguinal Ring:** Opening in the external oblique aponeurosis; the ring contains the ilioinguinal nerve and spermatic cord or round ligament.
   G. **Internal Ring:** Bordered superiorly by internal oblique muscle and inferomedially by the inferior epigastric vessels and the transversalis fascia.
   H. **Processus Vaginalis:** A diverticulum of peritoneum which descends with testicle, and lies adjacent to the spermatic cord. May enlarge to become the sac of an indirect inguinal hernia.
   I. **Femoral Canal:** Formed by the borders of the inguinal ligament, lacunar ligament, Cooper's ligament, and femoral sheath.

## III. Classification of Hernias
   A. **Indirect Inguinal Hernia:** Hernia sac is located anteromedial to the spermatic cord; the sac exits through the internal ring and lies lateral to the inferior epigastric artery. The indirect inguinal hernia is the most common inguinal hernia in either sex.
   B. **Direct Inguinal Hernia:** Hernia passes through Hasselbalch's triangle and lies medial to inferior epigastric artery.
   C. **Pantaloon Hernia:** Combination of both direct and indirect inguinal hernias.
   D. **Femoral Hernia:** Hernia passes through the femoral canal and lies medial to the femoral vein.
   E. **Umbilical Hernia:** Hernia passes through the umbilical ring. This hernia is usually congenital, but may be acquired, especially in patients with

ascites.
- F. **Incisional Hernia:** Hernia appears after surgery through a previous fascial closure.
- G. **Epigastric Hernia:** Caused by a defect in the linea alba, and located above umbilicus; frequently multiple.
- H. **Obturator Hernia:** Hernia passes through obturator foramen.
- I. **Spigelian Hernia:** Hernia occurring at semilunar line, at the lateral edge of the rectus muscle.
- J. **Petit's Hernia:** Hernia passes through lumbar triangle.
- K. **Perineal Hernia:** Hernia passes through a defect in the muscular pelvic floor; rectal prolapse often occurs.
- L. **Sciatic Hernia:** Hernia sac passes through greater or lesser sacrosciatic foramen; rarest type of hernias.

# Evaluation of the Hernia Patient

### I. Clinical Evaluation
- A. **History:** Patient complains of a soft mass that increases in size with straining. The mass may reduce manually or spontaneously. Pain may occur with straining. History of symptoms of small bowel obstruction may be present.
- B. Hernias may be caused by obesity, chronic cough, straining at stools due to constipation; straining at urination; ascites, previous abdominal surgery.
- C. **Physical Exam:** Palpable mass which increases in size when the patient strains; examine in the upright and supine positions; examine with patient relaxed and straining.
- D. **Examination for Hernias:** The examiner places index finger upward into scrotum, and into the external inguinal ring while patient strains or coughs. Direct hernias are felt on the medial side of the examiner's finger; indirect hernias are felt on the tip of the finger.
- E. Examine for prostatic enlargement and complete a rectal exam. Consider flexible sigmoidoscopy/colonoscopy.

# Surgical Repair Techniques for Hernias

### I. Surgical Techniques
- A. **Bassini Repair:** Approximation of conjoint tendon and the transversalis fascia to the edge of inguinal ligament.
- B. **McVay Repair (Cooper's Ligament Repair):** Approximation of conjoint tendon to Cooper's ligament; a relaxing incision in rectus sheath may be added.
- C. **Halsted Repair:** Same as Bassini repair, except imbricated external oblique is used to reinforce the repair beneath the spermatic cord.
- D. **Ligation of Sac:** Useful only in children who have only a simple patency of processus vaginalis.
- E. **Pre-Peritoneal Hernia Repair:** Hernia defect is exposed and repaired from beneath fascia in preperitoneal space.
- F. **Femoral Hernia Repair:** Use McVay or Cooper's ligament repair to repair femoral hernias. Do not attempt reduction of tender femoral hernias.

## 56 Hernia Repair Technique

   G. **Ventral Hernias:** Primary repair of fascial defect. Usually requires marlex mesh.
II. **Reduction of Incarcerated Hernias**
   A. Place patient in the Trendelenburg's position and sedate.
   B. Apply gentle continuous compression. No reduction should be attempted if possible strangulation. Strangulation is indicated by severe tenderness, induration, erythema, leukocytosis.
   C. Strangulated hernias should be treated in operating room. Do not attempt to reduce incarcerated femoral hernias.

# Hernia Repair Technique

I. **Indirect Hernia**
   A. Prep and draped the skin of the abdomen, inguinal region, upper thigh, and external genitalia. Place the incision 1 cm above and parallel to the inguinal ligament. Begin the incision at a point just above, and medial to, the pubic tubercle, and extend it to a point two-thirds the distance to the anterior iliac spine. Incise the subcutaneous fat in the length of the incision down to the external oblique aponeurosis. Clear the external oblique muscle of overlying fat and identify the external inguinal ring. Incise the aponeurosis of the external oblique, beginning laterally and splitting the aponeurosis in the direction of its fibers, taking care not to injure the underlying ilioinguinal nerve. Expose the inguinal canal in which the spermatic cord and the indirect inguinal hernia are located.
   B. Use blunt dissection to mobilize the spermatic cord and the associated hernia up to the level of the pubic tubercle. Lift these structures up from the floor of the inguinal canal, and encircle with a Penrose drain. Retract the drain anteriorly, and free the rest of the cord from the floor of the canal. Use sharp and blunt dissection to incise the anterior muscular and fascial investments of the cord.
   C. Sharply incise the internal spermatic fascia, and locate the hernial sac; identify the spermatic artery, venous plexus, and vas deferens before opening the sac.
   D. Incise the indirect hernial sac, anteriorly along its long axis, using caution if the sac is filled with small bowel or omentum. Place an index finger inside the hernial sac, and separate the sac from surrounding cord structures using sharp and blunt dissection. Carry dissection proximally to the internal inguinal ring.
   E. Close the sac with a circumferential purse-string suture on an atraumatic, gastrointestinal needle. Tie this suture, being careful that no abdominal organs are within the purse string (high ligation of the sac). Reinforce this ligation by placing another transfixion suture through the sac, 1 mm distal to the purse-string suture. Transect the sac a few millimeters below the second suture, and cut both sutures and allow sac to retract into the retroperitoneum. Remove the sac. Inspect the floor of the inguinal canal, and if there is only minimal dilation of the internal ring, the hernia repair can be completed by placing a few interrupted sutures at the medial border of the internal ring and completing a Bassini repair.
   F. If the hernia is moderately sized, use a modification of the Bassini repair. Place a series of interrupted sutures in the transversalis fascia beginning medially at the level of the pubic tubercle, and carry the sutures laterally

as far as the medial border of the internal ring. Incorporate the posterior fibers of the conjoint tendon, or use the posterior fascia of the transversalis abdominous muscle with some of the muscular fibers of the internal oblique muscle.
G. Begin suturing medially at Cooper's ligament, and transition at the femoral sheath to Poupart's ligament. Place the sutures 1 cm apart, and use nonabsorbable monofilament suture of 00 or heavier. Tie the sutures to reinforce the floor of the inguinal canal.
H. The reconstructed deep inguinal ring should be tight enough to prohibit protrusion of a new hernial sac without obstructing the blood supply of the cord or venous return of the testicle.
I. Replace the ilioinguinal nerve and the spermatic cord in the inguinal canal, and reapproximate the external oblique aponeurosis over the cord with interrupted, nonabsorbable, 000 sutures, taking care not to damage the underlying nerve or cord.
J. Close the subcutaneous tissues with interrupted, fine, absorbable sutures in Scarpa's fascia, and close the skin with staples or subcuticular sutures. Apply a sterile dressing.

## II. Surgical Repair of Direct Inguinal Hernias
A. The skin incision is the same as for repair of the indirect inguinal hernia. The direct inguinal hernia appears as a diffuse bulge in the area of Hesselbach's triangle, appreciated by palpating with a fingertip. Reduce the direct inguinal hernia bulging through Hesselbach's triangle with a series of interrupted, inverting, 00, nonabsorbable sutures placed in the redundant properitoneal fat. It is not necessary to provide high ligation and amputation of the hernial sac unless the sac is narrow-necked or diverticular, in which case the sac may be dealt with as described for the repair of the indirect hernia.
B. Repair the fascial defect in Hesselbach's triangle with a Cooper's ligament or modified McVay-type repair. Use sharp and blunt dissection of the floor of the inferior portion of the inguinal canal to expose the lacunar ligament and Cooper's ligament. Dissect laterally along Cooper's ligament as far as the medial aspect of the femoral vein. Make a relaxing incision in the deep portion of the anterior rectus sheath, then grasp the medial and superior edge of the defect in Hesselbach's triangle with Allis clamps.
C. Place a series of interrupted sutures, beginning medially at the pubic tubercle, and carry laterally as far as the femoral vein. Place these sutures first in the periosteum of the pubic tubercle, and then more laterally in Cooper's ligament itself. With the superior bite of the suture, catch the superior edge of the hernia defect. Place 4 to 8 sutures. Shift the suture line anteriorly, continuing the lateral portion of the repair by suturing the remaining portion of the superior edge of the defect in Hesselbach's triangle to the inguinal ligament ("transition" stitch).
D. Check the appropriate snugness of the deep inguinal ring. When all sutures are placed, tie the sutures medial to lateral. Check the hernia repair for sturdiness and for excessive tension on the sutures. Replace the cord and the ilioinguinal nerve in the bed of the inguinal canal, and reapproximate the external oblique aponeurosis over these structures. Close the subcutaneous tissue and skin, and apply a sterile dressing. Close the skin with microporous adhesive tape or a subcuticular suture.

# Hematemesis and Upper Gastrointestinal Bleeding

I. **Clinical Evaluation**
   A. Determine the duration of hematemesis (vomiting bright red blood or coffee ground material), volume of blood, recent hematocrit. Determine whether the bleeding occurred after forceful vomiting (Mallory-Weiss Syndrome).
   B. Abdominal pain, melena, hematochezia (bright red blood per rectum); history of peptic ulcer, esophagitis, prior bleeding episodes may be present.
   C. **Precipitating Factors:** Use of alcohol, aspirin, nonsteroidal anti-inflammatory agents, steroids, anticoagulants should be sought.
   D. **Past Testing or Treatment:** X-ray studies, endoscopy.
   E. The patient may have a past history of gastrointestinal bleeding; prior operations, cardiovascular disease, bleeding disorders.

II. **Physical Exam**
   A. **General:** Pallor, shallow rapid respirations; tachycardia indicates a 10% blood volume loss; postural hypotension with an increase pulse of 20 and a decrease in systolic of 20 indicates a 20-30% loss.
   B. **Skin:** Delayed capillary refill, pallor. Stigmata of liver disease: Jaundice, spider angiomas, parotid gland hypertrophy.
   C. **Chest:** Gynecomastia (cirrhosis).
   D. **Abdomen:** Scars, tenderness, masses, hepatomegaly; dilated abdominal veins. Stool gross or occult blood.
   E. Depressed mental status.

III. **Laboratory Evaluation**
   A. CBC, SMA 12, liver function tests, amylase, PT/PTT, type and cross PRBC, FFP. CBC q6h.
   B. EKG, UA. CXR, upright abdomen (evaluate for free air under the diaphragm).

IV. **Differential Diagnosis of Upper Bleeding:** Peptic ulcer, gastritis, esophageal varices, Mallory Weiss tear (gastroesophageal junction tear because of vomiting or retching), esophagitis, swallowed blood from epistaxis, malignancy (esophageal, gastric), angiodysplasias, aorto-enteric fistula, hematobilia.

V. **Diagnostic and Therapeutic Approach to Upper Gastrointestinal Bleeding**
   A. If the bleeding appears to have stopped or has significantly slowed, medical therapy with H2 blockers, and saline lavage is usually all that is required. The diagnostic and therapeutic approach is based on an estimate of the volume and duration of blood loss, and on the patient's clinical history.
   B. Place a minimum of two 14-16 gauge IV lines. Administer 1-2 liters of normal saline solution until blood is ready, then transfuse PRBC's as fast as possible; estimate blood transfusion requirement based on blood loss rate, vital signs (typically 2-6 units PRBC's are needed). Administer type O negative blood in emergent situations. If hypotensive consider endotracheal intubation.
   C. For each 3 units of PRBC transfused, calcium chloride (1 gm IV over an

hour) is given to prevent transfusion hypocalcemia.
- D. Rapidly assess the patient's need for surgical intervention. Central venous monitoring or pulmonary artery catheter monitoring is necessary in the presence of hypotension or hypoxemia.
- E. Place a large bore nasogastric tube, then lavage with 2 L of room temperature tap water, then connect to low intermittent suction, repeat lavage q1h.
- F. Administer oxygen by nasal cannula, guided by pulse oximetry. Foley to closed drainage. Keep patient NPO.
- G. Record volume and character of lavage. The NG tube may be removed when bleeding is no longer active.
- H. If bright red blood is present in nasogastric tube aspirate, lavage with room temperature saline to remove blood clots.
- I. Check serial hematocrits, and maintain greater than 30 vol%. Monitor for coagulopathy and correct if necessary with fresh frozen plasma. Consider pulmonary artery catheterization (Swan-Ganz) to assess effectiveness of resuscitation.
- J. Definitive diagnosis requires upper endoscopy at which time electrocoagulation of bleeding sites may be completed.

## VI. Mallory-Weiss Syndrome
- A. This disorder is defined as a mucosal tear at the gastroesophageal junction. It frequently follows violent retching and vomiting.
- B. Treatment is supportive, and the majority of patients stop bleeding spontaneously. Endoscopic coagulation or operative suturing may rarely be necessary.

## VII. Medical Treatment of Peptic Ulcers or Non-ulcer dyspepsia
- A. Ranitidine (Zantac) 50 mg IV bolus, then continuous infusion at 6.25-12.5 mg/h [150-300 mg in 250 mL D5W over 24h (11 cc/h)], or 50 mg IV q6-8h **OR**
- B. Cimetidine (Tagamet) 300 mg IV bolus, then continuous infusion at 37.5-50 mg/h (900 mg in 250 mL D5W over 24h), or 300 mg IV q6-8h **OR**
- C. Famotidine (Pepcid) 20 mg IV q12h.

**References:** See page 106.

# Variceal Bleeding

Hemorrhage from esophageal and gastric varices is a severe complication of chronic liver disease.

## I. Clinical Evaluation
- A. Variceal bleeding should be considered in any patient who presents with significant upper gastrointestinal bleeding, because some patients with liver disease do not exhibit the classic signs of cirrhosis (eg, spider angiomas, palmar erythema, leukonychia, clubbing, parotid enlargement, Dupuytren's contracture).
- B. When patients present with jaundice, lower extremity edema and ascites, the diagnosis of decompensated liver disease is obvious.
- C. The severity of the bleeding episode can be assessed on the basis of the presence of orthostatic changes (eg, resting tachycardia, postural hypotension), which indicates that about one third or more of blood volume has been lost.

## 60 Variceal bleeding

   D. If the patient's sensorium is altered because of hepatic encephalopathy, the risk of aspiration mandates endotracheal intubation.
   E. Placement of a large-caliber nasogastric tube (22 F or 24 F) permits lavage for removal of blood and clots in preparation for endoscopy.
   F. Lavage should be performed with tap water, because saline may contribute to retention of sodium and water.

## II. Resuscitation
   A. Blood should be replaced as soon as possible. While blood for transfusion is being made available, intravascular volume should be replenished with intravenous albumin in isotonic saline solution (Albuminar-5) or normal saline solution if the patient does not have ascites or evidence of decompensation.
   B. Once euvolemia is established, intravenous infusion should be changed to solutions with a lower sodium content (5% dextrose with 1/2 or 1/4 normal saline).
   C. Fresh frozen plasma is administered for patients who have been given massive transfusions because of the "washout" phenomenon; in such cases, calcium should also be replaced. FFP is also indicated for patients with coagulopathy.
   D. Blood should be transfused to maintain a hematocrit of at least 25%. Serial hematocrit estimations during continued bleeding are done to determine whether replacement is adequate. Values may, however, be inaccurate after acute blood loss.

## III. Treatment of Variceal Hemorrhage
   A. Pharmacologic Agents
      1. **Octreotide (Sandostatin)** 50 mcg IV over 5-10 min, followed by 50 mcg/h for 48 hours (1200 mcg in 250 mL D5W); somatostatin analog; beneficial in controlling hemorrhage.
      2. **Vasopressin (Pitressin)**, a posterior pituitary hormone, causes splanchnic arteriolar vasoconstriction and reduction in portal pressure.
         a. Dosage is 20 units IV over 20-30 min, then 0.2-0.4 units/minute; complications increase with dosages of 0.4 to 0.6 U/min (100 U in 250 mL D5W).
         b. Concomitant use of transdermal nitroglycerin, 0.4 mg/hr for 12 hours may reduce portal pressure by about 10%. This agent mitigates the vasoconstrictor effects of vasopressin on the myocardial and splanchnic circulations.
   B. Additional treatments should be considered if bleeding continues, as indicated by fresh blood aspirate from the nasogastric tube and the need for continued blood transfusion (2-3 U of packed cells every 8 hours after start of infusion).
   C. Tamponade Devices
      1. Bleeding from varices can be reduced with the use of tamponade balloon tubes. However, the benefit is temporary, and prolonged tamponade causes severe esophageal ulceration.
      2. The Linton-Nachlas tube is recommended; it has a gastric balloon and several ports in the esophageal component. The tube is kept in place for 6 to 12 hours while preparations for endoscopic or radiologic treatment are being made.
   D. Endoscopic Management of Bleeding Varices
      1. Endoscopic sclerotherapy involves injection of a sclerosant solution into varices during endoscopy. The success of the treatment is

enhanced by repeating treatments at weekly intervals or less often.
2. **Endoscopic variceal ligation** involves placement of tiny rubber bands on varices during endoscopy.
   a. There are fewer complications with ligation than with sclerotherapy, and bleeding and mortality rates are lower.
   b. Ligation is the preferred treatment when varices are large and there is no active bleeding.

E. **Surgery**
   1. Portal-systemic shunt surgery the most definitive therapy for bleeding varices. The placement of a shunt creates an anastomosis between portal and systemic veins, allowing decompression of the hypertensive portal venous system and almost complete elimination of rebleeding. However, some of the procedures have a 30-40% rate of hepatic encephalopathy, and there is no difference in survival rates between shunt surgery and medical treatments.
   2. Shunts that preserve protal blood flow are preferred, such as the distal splenorenal and the small-diameter portacaval H-graft shunts.

F. **Transjugular Intrahepatic Portacaval Shunt (TIPS)**
   1. Under fluoroscopy, a needle is advanced into the liver through the internal jugular and hepatic veins, and inserted into a large branch of the portal vein. A balloon is then used to enlarge the track to permit the placement of a stent.
   2. Because TIPS is a shunt procedure, encephalopathy occurs in about 35% of patients and occlusion, which can occur in 50% of patients, of the stent may cause recurrent variceal bleeding.

IV. **Approach to Treatment of Variceal Hemorrhage**
   A. Patients initially should be given octreotide (Sandostatin) or vasopressin infusion and transdermal nitroglycerin while awaiting endoscopic treatment.
   B. If bleeding is not brisk and varices are large, endoscopic ligation is preferred; for active bleeding from a spurting varix, sclerotherapy is best.
   C. Treatment failure warrants the use of a portal-systemic shunt in good risk patients.
   D. Liver transplantation should be considered poor-risk patients and when other therapy fails.

**References:** See page 106.

# Peptic Ulcer Disease

I. **Clinical Evaluation**
   A. Peptic ulcer disease (PUD) is characterized by epigastric pain that may be exacerbated by fasting and relieved by food or antacids. Nausea and vomiting are common. Hematemesis ("coffee ground" emesis) or melena (black tarry stools) are indicative of significant bleeding.
   B. **Physical Examination.** Tenderness to deep palpation is often present in the epigastrium; stool is often guaiac-positive.
   C. Helicobacter pylori (HP) is the most frequent cause of PUD. Nonsteroidal anti-inflammatory drugs (NSAIDs), smoking, alcohol, and pathologically high acid-secreting states (Zollinger-Ellison syndrome) are less common causes.
   D. All patients with PUD and documented HP infection should be treated for

## 62 Peptic Ulcer Disease

      HP during an active ulceration or while asymptomatic.
- **E.** Treatment of HP in patients with PUD significantly decreases the recurrence rate of PUD and virtually eliminates the need for maintenance therapy with acid-suppressive medications.

### II. Detection of Helicobacter Pylori Infection
- **A.** Patients with symptoms of uncomplicated PUD should be evaluated with a non-endoscopic serologic antibody test for HP. Patients with complicated disease (eg, age >50, severe pain, upper GI bleeding) should receive endoscopy and biopsy for HP.
- **B. Non-endoscopic Tests (non-invasive)**
  1. Serologic testing for antibodies to HP (IgG and IgA), by ELISA quantitation or by immunoassay, has good sensitivity and specificity. These tests are used for initial screening; however, they are not useful to confirm eradication. The immunoassay is an easy to perform office procedure.
  2. **Labeled Urea Breath Tests.** $^{13}C$-urea and $^{14}C$-urea breath tests have high sensitivity and high specificity and are easy to perform in the office. They are useful, non-invasive tests to confirm eradication of HP 4 weeks after the completion of therapy.
- **C. Endoscopic Tests**
  1. Rapid urease tests (CLOtest, Pyloritek) have good sensitivity and specificity. The results are usually rapidly available.
  2. **Histologic Examination** give additional information about the degree of underlying inflammation or other mucosal abnormalities.
  3. **Culture** requires a microbiology lab with adequate experience. It is not usually needed except to check for resistant organisms.
- **D. Eradication** is usually assessed clinically by alleviation of symptoms. If symptoms recur, a urea breath test or endoscopic biopsy may be useful to confirm eradication.

### III. Treatment of Peptic Ulcer Disease
- **A. Active Ulcer.** For patients with an active duodenal or gastric ulcer, acid suppression with a histamine-2 receptor antagonist or proton pump inhibitor is continued for a total of 4 to 8 weeks, with anti-HP therapy for the first 2 weeks.
- **B. Treatment Regimens for Elimination of H. pylori**
  1. One week of therapy is recommended
  2. **Bismuth, Metronidazole, Tetracycline, Ranitidine**
     - a. 14 day therapy.
     - b. Bismuth (PeptoBismol) 2 tablets po qid.
     - c. Metronidazole (Flagyl) 250 mg po qid (tid if cannot tolerate the qid dosing).
     - d. Tetracycline 500 mg po qid (amoxicillin 500 mg po qid in children).
     - e. Ranitidine (Zantac) 150 mg PO bid.
     - f. Efficacy is greater than 90%; very inexpensive, proven efficacy in multiple studies, and moderate side-effects. Tetracycline is better than amoxicillin unless contraindicated.
  3. **Amoxicillin, Omeprazole, Clarithromycin (AOC)**
     - a. 10 days of therapy.
     - b. Amoxicillin 1 gm po bid.
     - c. Omeprazole (Prilosec) 20 mg po bid.
     - d. Clarithromycin (Biaxin) 500 mg po bid.
     - e. Expensive, but usually well tolerated.

## Peptic Ulcer Disease

### 4. Metronidazole, Omeprazole, Clarithromycin (MOC)
   a. 10 days of therapy
   b. Metronidazole 500 mg po bid.
   c. Omeprazole (Prilosec) 20 mg po bid.
   d. Clarithromycin 500 mg po bid.
   e. Efficacy is >80%
   f. Expensive, usually well tolerated.

### C. Omeprazole, Clarithromycin (OC)
   1. 14 days of therapy.
   2. Omeprazole (Prilosec) 40 mg po qd for 14 days, then 20 mg qd for and additional 14 days of therapy.
   3. Clarithromycin 500 mg po tid.

### D. Ranitidine-Bismuth-Citrate, Clarithromycin (Rbc-C)
   1. 14 days of therapy.
   2. Ranitidine-bismuth-citrate (Tritec) 400 mg po bid.
   3. Clarithromycin 500 mg po tid.
   4. Efficacy is 70-80%; expensive

### E. Follow-up Evaluation.
At least 4 weeks after completion of treatment, confirmation of HP eradication consists of a urea breath test or repeat endoscopy.

### F. Acute $H_2$-Blocker Therapy
   1. Cimetidine (Tagamet), 400 mg bid or 800 mg hs.
   2. Ranitidine (Zantac), 150 mg bid or 300 mg hs.
   3. Famotidine (Pepcid), 20 mg bid or 40 mg hs
   4. Nizatidine (Axid Pulvules), 150 mg bid or 300 mg hs
   5. Side effects are uncommon.
   6. Maintenance therapy is one half of the therapeutic dose. If H. pylori therapy has been completed, most ulcers will not recur, and maintenance therapy will not be required.

### G. Mucosal Protective Agent--Sucralfate (Carafate)
is a mucosal, protective agent; 1 gm tid, before meals and hs; constipation is common; binds to other drugs.

### H. Proton Pump Inhibitors
   1. Omeprazole (Prilosec) is reserved for ulcers that are refractory to $H_2$ blockers and sucralfate. 20 mg qd. Side effects are rare.
   2. Lansoprazole (Prevacid). 15 mg before breakfast qd.

## IV. Surgical Treatment of Peptic Ulcer Disease

### A. Indications for Surgery.
Exsanguinating hemorrhage, >5 units transfusion in 24-hours, rebleeding during same hospitalization; intractability, perforation, gastric outlet obstruction, endoscopic signs predictive of rebleeding.

### B. Emergency Surgery for Peptic Ulcer Disease
   1. **Unstable Patients** should receive a truncal vagotomy, oversewing of bleeding ulcer bed, and a pyloroplasty.
   2. **Stable Patients** should be managed with oversewing of the ulcer bed with either a vagotomy and antrectomy or a proximal gastric vagotomy.

### C. Surgical Therapy of Duodenal Ulcer Disease
   1. **Operative Therapy.** If the ulcer is still active after adequate medical therapy, surgery should be considered.
   2. **Vagotomy Procedures**
      a. Truncal vagotomy with drainage procedure (pyloroplasty or gastrojejunostomy).

b. Selective vagotomy with drainage procedure.
   c. Proximal gastric (parietal cell, highly selective) vagotomy (usually without drainage procedure).
   3. **Vagotomy and Antrectomy** with gastroduodenostomy (Billroth I) or gastrojejunostomy (Billroth II). Antrectomy consists of removal of distal one third of stomach.
   D. **Surgical Therapy for Gastric Ulcer** consists of gastric resection to include ulcer. Vagotomy should be added in patients with increased acid secretion.

**References:** See page 106.

# Lower Gastrointestinal Bleeding

The spontaneous remission rate for lower gastrointestinal bleeding, even with massive bleeding, is 80% (the same as for upper gastrointestinal bleeding). No source of bleeding can be identified in 12%, and bleeding is recurrent in 25%:

Bleeding has usually ceased by the time the patient presents to the emergency room, although copious amounts of blood and clots may continue to be passed from the rectum.

I. **Initial Clinical Evaluation**
   A. The severity of blood loss and hemodynamic status should be assessed immediately. Initial management consists of resuscitation with colloidal solutions (hetastarch [Hespan]) or crystalloid solutions (lactated Ringers solution) and with blood products if necessary.
   B. An initial diagnostic evaluation, to determine the source of bleeding, is performed while the patient is being resuscitated.
   C. The duration and quantity of bleeding are assessed; however, the duration of bleeding is often underestimated and the quantity is often overestimated.
   D. Risk factors that may have contributed to the bleeding should be assessed, such as the use of nonsteroidal anti-inflammatory drugs, anticoagulants, history of colonic diverticulosis, renal failure, coagulopathy, colonic polyps, hemorrhoids, chemotherapy or radiotherapy.
   E. **Hematochezia.** Bright red or maroon blood per rectum suggests a lower GI source; 11-20% of patients with an upper GI bleed will have hematochezia as a result of rapid blood loss (these patients are usually in shock).
   F. **Melena.** Sticky, black, foul-smelling stools suggest a source proximal to the ligament of Treitz, but can result from bleeding in the small intestine or proximal colon. Iron and bismuth can turn stools black but not melanotic (shiny and tarry).
   G. **Malignancy** may be indicated by a change in stool caliber, anorexia, weight loss and malaise.
   H. Patients may have a history of hemorrhoids, diverticulosis, inflammatory bowel disease, peptic ulcer, gastritis, cirrhosis or esophageal varices.
   I. **Associated Findings**
      1. **Abdominal pain** may result from ischemic bowel, inflammatory bowel disease, or a ruptured aortic aneurysm.
      2. **Painless, massive bleeding** often indicates vascular bleeding from

# Lower Gastrointestinal Bleeding

      diverticula, angiodysplasia or hemorrhoids.
3. **Bloody diarrhea** suggests inflammatory bowel disease or an infectious origin.
4. **Bleeding with rectal pain** is seen with anal fissures, hemorrhoids, and rectal ulcers.
5. **Chronic constipation** suggests hemorrhoidal bleeding; new onset constipation or thin stools suggests a left-sided colonic malignancy.
6. **Blood on the toilet paper or dripping** into the toilet water after a bowel movement suggests a perianal source.
7. **Blood coating the outside of stool** suggests a lesion in the anal canal.
8. **Blood streaking or mixed in with the stool** may result from a polyp or malignancy in the descending colon.
9. **Maroon colored stools** often indicate small bowel and proximal colon bleeding.

## II. Physical Examination
   A. **Postural Hypotension** suggests a 20% blood volume loss; whereas, overt signs of shock (pallor, hypotension, and tachycardia) indicate a 30-40% blood loss.
   B. The skin may be cool and pale with delayed capillary refill if bleeding has been significant.
   C. Stigmata of liver disease including jaundice, caput medusae, gynecomastia, and palmar erythema should be sought since these patients frequently have GI bleeding.

## III. Approach to the Diagnosis of Lower Gastrointestinal Bleeding
   A. Rapid clinical evaluation and resuscitation should precede diagnostic or therapeutic studies. Intravenous fluids (1-2 liters) should be infused over 10-20 minutes to restore intravascular volume, and blood is transfused if there is rapid ongoing blood loss or if hypotension or tachycardia is present. Coagulopathy is corrected with fresh frozen plasma or platelets.
   B. When small amounts of bright red blood are passed per rectum, the lower gastrointestinal tract can be assumed to be the source.
   C. In patients with large-volume maroon stools, nasogastric tube aspiration should be performed to exclude massive upper gastrointestinal hemorrhage. Occult blood testing of lavage fluid is useless because mild trauma from tube placement may cause a positive result.
   D. If the nasogastric aspirate contains no blood, then anoscopy and sigmoidoscopy should be performed to determine whether a colonic mucosal abnormality (ischemic or infectious colitis) or hemorrhoids might be the cause of bleeding.
   E. If these measures fail to yield a diagnosis, rapid administration of polyethylene glycol-electrolyte solution (CoLyte or GoLYTELY) should be initiated orally or by means of a nasogastric tube; 4 L of the lavage solution is given over a 2- to 3-hour period. This allows diagnostic and therapeutic colonoscopy and adequately prepares the bowel should emergency operation become necessary.

## IV. Causes of Lower Gastrointestinal Bleeding
   A. Angiodysplasia and diverticular disease of the right colon account for the vast majority of episodes of acute lower gastrointestinal bleeding.
   B. Most acute LGI bleeding originates from the colon; however, 15-20% of episodes arise from the small intestine and the upper gastrointestinal tract.

- C. **Elderly Patients.** Diverticulosis and angiodysplasia are the most common causes of lower GI bleeding.
- D. **Younger Patients.** Hemorrhoids, anal fissures, and inflammatory bowel disease (IBD) are more common causes.
- E. **Angiodysplasia**
    1. Angiodysplastic lesions are small vascular tufts that are formed by capillaries, veins, and venules.
    2. Angiodysplastic lesions are commonly noted during colonoscopy, appearing as red dots or spider-like lesions 2 to 10 mm in diameter.
    3. Angiodysplastic lesions develop secondary, to chronic colonic distention, which leads to obstruction of venules.
    4. Angiodysplastic lesions are associated with advanced age, and they have a prevalence rate of 25% in elderly patients These lesions have also been associated with chronic renal failure, CREST syndrome, Rendu-Osler-Weber syndrome, and cirrhosis. Their association with aortic stenosis remains to be established.
    5. Even though angiodysplasia may be present throughout the entire colon, the most common site of bleeding remains the right colon. Most patients with angiodysplasia have recurrent minor bleeding; however, massive bleeding is not uncommon.
- F. **Diverticular Disease**
    1. Diverticular disease is the most common cause of acute lower gastrointestinal bleeding.
    2. 60% to 80% of bleeding diverticula are located in the right colon.
    3. 90% of all diverticula are found in the left colon.
    4. Diverticular bleeding tends to be massive, but it stops spontaneously in 80% of patients with only supportive care, and the rate of rebleeding is only 25%.

## V. Definitive Management of Lower GI Bleeding

- A. **Colonoscopy**
    1. Colonoscopy is the procedure of choice for diagnosing colonic causes of gastrointestinal bleeding. It should be performed after adequate preparation of the bowel, which permits identification of 80% of all causative colonic lesions. If the bowel cannot be adequately prepared because of persistent, acute bleeding, a bleeding scan or angiography is preferable.
    2. Endoscopy may be therapeutic for angiodysplastic lesions, polyps, and tumors, which can be effectively coagulated.
    3. If colonoscopy fails to reveal a source for the bleeding, the patient should be observed, since in about 80% of cases, bleeding ceases spontaneously.
- B. **Bleeding Scan**
    1. The technetium-labeled ("tagged") red blood cell bleeding scan can detect bleeding sites when bleeding is intermittent.
    2. If the result is positive, the next step is colonoscopy or angiography.
- C. **Angiography**
    1. Selective mesenteric angiography detects arterial bleeding that occurs at a rate of 0.5 mL/min or faster.
    2. Diverticular bleeding classically causes pooling of contrast medium within a specific diverticulum (extravasation).
    3. Bleeding angiodysplastic lesions demonstrate abnormal vasculature.
    4. Bleeding from angiodysplastic lesions usually is slow and rarely

necessitates therapeutic intervention. However, when active bleeding is seen with diverticular disease or angiodysplasia, selective arterial infusion of vasopressin is effective in arresting hemorrhage in 90%.

### D. Evaluation of the Small Bowel
1. If bleeding persists but no source is noted, the small bowel must be considered as a possible source.
2. The preferred technique for evaluating the small bowel is push enteroscopy (with an overtube) in combination with enteroclysis barium study.
3. Meckel's diverticulum, which usually presents in younger patients, is a common site of bleeding in the small intestine. The diagnosis can be confirmed by radionuclide Meckel's scanning, which identifies the ectopic gastric mucosa.

### E. Surgery
1. If bleeding continues and no source has been found, surgical intervention is warranted.
2. Surgical resection may be indicated for patients with recurrent diverticular bleeding, or for patients who have had persistent bleeding from colonic angiodysplasia and have required blood transfusions.
3. Treatment of lower gastrointestinal bleeding involves resection of the involved segment--for example, a right hemicolectomy or sigmoid resection. Patients with a diffuse process, such as ulcerative colitis, require a total proctocolectomy with ileostomy.
4. When laparotomy fails to identify a definitive source of bleeding, intraoperative endoscopy may be a useful adjunct.

## VI. Colon Polyps and Colon Cancers
**A.** These rarely cause significant acute LGI hemorrhage.
**B.** Left-sided and rectal neoplasms are more likely to cause gross bleeding than right sided lesions. Right sided lesions are more likely to cause anemia and occult bleeding.
**C. Diagnosis.** Colonoscopy.
**D. Treatment.** Colonoscopic excision or surgical resection.

## VII. Inflammatory Bowel Disease
**A.** Ulcerative colitis can occasionally cause severe GI bleeding associated with abdominal pain and diarrhea.
**B. Diagnosis.** Colonoscopy and biopsy.
**C. Treatment.** Medical treatment of the underlying disease; operation is required on rare occasions.

## VIII. Ischemic Colitis
**A.** This disorder is seen in elderly patients with known vascular disease; abdominal pain may be postprandial, and is associated with bloody diarrhea or rectal bleeding. Severe blood loss is unusual but can occur.
**B. Diagnosis.** Abdominal films may reveal "thumbprinting", caused by submucosal edema. Colonoscopy reveals a well-demarcated area of hyperemia, edema, and mucosal ulcerations. The splenic flexure and descending colon are the most common sites.
**C. Treatment:** Most episodes resolve spontaneously; however, vascular bypass or resection may be required.

## IX. Hemorrhoids
**A.** Hemorrhoids rarely cause massive acute blood loss. In patients with portal hypertension, rectal varices must be sought.
**B. Diagnosis.** Anoscopy and sigmoidoscopy.

**C. Treatment.** High fiber diet, stool softeners, or hemorrhoidectomy.

# Anorectal Disorders

## I. Hemorrhoids
  A. Hemorrhoids are dilated veins located beneath the lining of the anal canal.
  B. Internal hemorrhoids are located in the upper anal canal. External hemorrhoids are located in the lower anal canal.

## II. Internal Hemorrhoids
  A. Internal hemorrhoids become symptomatic when constipation causes disruption of the supporting tissues and resultant prolapse and excessive of the vascular anal cushions.
  B. The most common symptom of internal hemorrhoids is painless rectal bleeding, which is usually bright red and ranges from a few drops to a spattering stream at the end of defecation.
  C. If internal hemorrhoids remain prolapsed, a dull aching may occur.
  D. Blood and mucus stains may appear on underwear, and itching in the perianal region is common.

**Classification of Internal Hemorrhoids**

| Grade | Description | Symptoms |
|---|---|---|
| 1 | Non-prolapsing | Minimal bleeding |
| 2 | Prolapse with straining, reduce when spontaneously prolapsed | Bleeding, discomfort, pruritus |
| 3 | Prolapse with straining, manual reduction require when prolapsed | Bleeding, discomfort, pruritus |
| 4 | Cannot be reduced when prolapsed | Bleeding, discomfort, pruritus |

  E. **Management of Internal Hemorrhoids**
   1. **Grade 1 and uncomplicated grade 2 hemorrhoids** are treated with avoidance of nonsteroidal anti-inflammatory drugs and dietary modification (increased fiber and fluids and avoidance of binding, spicy, and fatty foods).
   2. **Symptomatic grade 2 and grade 3 hemorrhoids**
      a. Treatment consists of hemorrhoid banding. An anoscope is used to place a rubber band ligature above and around the hemorrhoid. The tissue sloughs in about a week, leaving an ulcer. Two or three bandings at separate visits are often required.

- **b.** Major complications are rare and consist of excessive pain, bleeding, and infection. Discomfort after banding is usually relieved by warm baths and oral analgesics.
- **3. Grade 4 hemorrhoids** require surgical hemorrhoidectomy.

## III. External Hemorrhoids
- **A.** External hemorrhoids occur most often in young and middle-aged adults, becoming symptomatic only when they become thrombosed.
- **B.** External hemorrhoids are characterized by rapid onset of constant burning or throbbing pain accompanying a new rectal lump. Bluish skin-covered lumps are visible at the anal verge.
- **C.** Pain is maximal in the first 48 hours and decreases thereafter to minimal discomfort after the 4 days.
- **D. Management of External Hemorrhoids**
  1. If patients are seen in the first 48 hours, the entire lesion can be excised in the office. Local anesthetic is infiltrated, and the thrombus and overlying skin are excised with scissors. The resulting wound heals by secondary intention.
  2. If thrombosis occurred more than 48 hours prior, spontaneous resolution should be permitted to occur; symptoms may be relieved by pain medication, sitz baths, and stool softeners. Thrombosed external hemorrhoids may erode through the skin, leading to hematochezia. The problem requires only direct pressure for hemostasis.

## IV. Anal Fissures
- **A.** Anal fissures are linear ulcers that extend from just below the dentate line to the anal verge, occurring most often in young and middle-aged adults but can they affect all ages.
- **B.** These lesions are most common in the posterior midline, but they may in the anterior midline in 10%. Chronic lesions can cause a skin tag at the outermost edge (the sentinel pile).
- **C.** Chronic fissures can undergo suppuration and extend into the surrounding tissues, causing a perianal abscess.
- **D.** Trauma to the anal canal during defecation is the cause of anal fissures.
- **E.** Anal fissures cause a tearing anal pain during defecation and gnawing or throbbing discomfort after defecation. Any bleeding is usually slight.
- **F.** Anal fissures are confirmed by inspection of the anus.
- **G. Treatment of Anal Fissures**
  1. **Medical management:**
     - **a.** Bulking fiber supplements together with warm sitz baths and a high-fiber diet are the most effective treatment methods.
     - **b.** Topical medication and suppositories are not effective when used alone but are not harmful.
  2. **Lateral Partial Internal Sphincterotomy**
     - **a.** This procedure is indicated when medical therapy fails. It consists of surgical division of a portion of the internal sphincter, and it is highly effective in relieving pain.
     - **b. Adverse effects** include incontinence to flatus and seepage.

## V. Perianal Abscess
- **A.** The anal glands, located in the base of the anal crypts at the level of the dentate line, are the most common source of perianal infection.
- **B.** Acute infection presents as an abscess, and chronic infection results in

a fistula. Infections start in the intersphincteric plane and can extend upward, downward, and circumferentially around the anus.

- C. The most common symptoms of perianal abscess are swelling and pain that is throbbing, continuous, and progressive. Fevers and chills may occur. Perianal abscess is common in diabetic and immunosuppressed patients, and there is often a history of chronic constipation or previous abscesses.
- D. A tender mass with fluctuant characteristics or induration is apparent on rectal exam.
- E. **Management of Perianal Abscess**
    1. A perianal abscess is treated with incision and drainage. Antibiotic therapy alone is not adequate. If the abscess is small, incision and drainage as an office procedure using a local anesthetic is usually possible. Large abscesses require regional or general anesthesia for adequate drainage.
    2. A cruciate incision is made close to the anal verge and the corners are excised to create an elliptical opening, which promotes drainage.
    3. An Antibiotic effective against bowel flora, such as Zosyn, Timentin, or Cefotetan, is used.
- F. An anorectal abscess can progress readily to Fournier's gangrene (necrotizing fasciitis of the perineum and abdominal wall), especially in diabetic or immunocompromised patients. This life-threatening condition requires immediate, radical debridement.
- G. About half of patients with anorectal abscesses will develop a fistula tract between the anal glands and the perianal mucosa, known as a fistula-in-ano, which manifests as either incomplete healing of the drainage site or recurrence. All patients with anorectal abscess should be reexamined 4 weeks after treatment to determine if a fistula has formed. Permanent healing of a fistula-in-ano requires a surgical fistulotomy.

## VI. Condylomata Acuminata

- A. Condylomata acuminata, or genital warts, are a common venereal disease caused by the human papillomavirus. They are spread by intimate contact, including autoinoculation, and have an incubation period that ranges from weeks to months.
- B. An estimated 1% of sexually active adults have visible lesions. Several subtypes of human papillomaviruses are associated with malignancy.
- C. Patients with small lesions usually have few symptoms. Bleeding, discharge, itching, and pain may occur. Warts appear pink or white with a papilliform surface.
- D. **Treatment of Condylomata**
    1. Topical caustic agents, such as podophyllum resin or trichloroacetic acid, work best on small lesions when applied repetitively.
    2. Lesions that are persistent despite topical treatment, extensive, or that extend into the anal canal are managed with surgical ablation.
    3. Recurrence is common.

# Fistula-in-Ano

### I. Clinical Evaluation
  A. A fistula-in-ano develops when an anorectal abscess forms a fistula between the anal canal and the perianal skin. The fistula may develop after an anorectal abscess has been drained operatively, or the fistula may develop spontaneously; less commonly, inflammatory bowel disease may cause a fistula-in-ano.
  B. The fistula is characterized by persistent purulent or feculent drainage, soiling the underwear.
  C. The fistula orifice can be seen peripheral to the anal verge. Complex fistulae may have multiple tracts with multiple orifices ("pepper-pot anus").

### II. Treatment of Fistula-in-Ano
  A. Fistulae will not resolve without definitive treatment. The more common type of fistula, located at the anorectal junction, has an external opening where it can be drained operatively. The entire epithelialized tract must be found and obliterated.
  B. Goodsall's rule predicts the course of simple fistulae that exit the skin within 3 cm of the anal verge. Anterior fistulae go straight toward the anorectal junction; posterior fistulae follow a curving course toward the posterior midline and enter the anorectal junction.
  C. Occasionally, it can be difficult to distinguish a pilonidal cyst-sinus (coccygeal region) from a fistula-in-ano. Probing the tract under anesthesia usually will reveal its origin.
  D. **Fistulotomy.** For fistulae that do not cross both internal and external sphincters, the tract should be unroofed and curetted. The lesion should then be allowed to heal by secondary intention.
  E. **Fistulectomy.** Deeper fistulae should be treated by coring out the epithelialized tract to its origin; however, the fistula may recur.
  F. **Seton Procedure.** Complex fistulae or fistulae that traverse the sphincter can be treated by looping a heavy suture through the entire tract under tension. The suture should be tightened weekly until it "cuts" gradually to the surface, the tract will heal gradually behind the suture.
  G. **Palliative Colostomy:** Extremely severe fistulization throughout the perineum may require fecal diversion for symptomatic relief.

# Colorectal Cancer

### I. Clinical Evaluation of Colorectal Cancer
  A. Colorectal cancer is the second most common solid malignancy in adults and the second leading cause of cancer death in the U.S.
  B. Flexible sigmoidoscopy for screening is indicated for asymptomatic, healthy adults over age 50. All adults with anemia or guaiac positive stools must be evaluated for colorectal cancer in the absence of other causes; older adults (>40) should be evaluated even if other sources of bleeding have been found. Hemorrhoids and cancer can coexist.
  C. Flexible sigmoidoscopy plus air contrast barium enema is adequate to evaluate the colon when the source of bleeding is thought to be benign anorectal disease.
  D. Total colonoscopy should be performed for any adult with gross or occult

rectal bleeding and no apparent anorectal source.
- **E.** Left sided or rectal lesions are characterized by blood streaked stools, change in caliber or consistency of stools, obstipation, alternating diarrhea and constipation, tenesmus (involuntary sphincter spasm during defecation).
- **F.** Right sided lesions are characterized by a triad of iron deficiency anemia, a right lower quadrant mass, and weakness.
- **G.** Cancers occasionally present as a large bowel obstruction, perforation or abscess.

## II. Laboratory Evaluation
- **A.** CBC with indices (hypochromic, microcytic anemia). Liver function tests may sometimes be elevated in metastatic disease.
- **B. Carcinoembryonic antigen (CEA):** Carcinoembryonic antigen is not a screening test; may be elevated in colorectal cancer but it is a nonspecific test (also elevated in other malignancies, some inflammatory bowel disease, cigarette smokers, and some normal persons). Valuable in monitoring the response to treatment and as a marker for recurrence or metastases requiring adjuvant therapy. Should be obtained prior to resection of the tumor and at intervals postoperatively.
- **C.** Colorectal cancer is detected by total colonoscopy with biopsies. Barium enema may complement colonoscopy since BE shows the exact anatomic location of the tumor. A chest X-ray should be done to search for metastases to the lungs.

## III. Management of Colorectal Carcinoma
- **A.** Surgical resection is indicated for colorectal adenocarcinoma, regardless of stage. Resection of the primary lesion prevents obstruction or perforation.
- **B.** Extremely advanced rectal lesions, which are not resectable, may be candidates for palliative radiation and a diverting colostomy.
- **C.** The extent of resection is determined by the relationship of the lesion to the lymphatic drainage and blood supply of the colon.
    1. **Cecum or Right Colon.** Right hemicolectomy.
    2. **Hepatic Flexure.** Extended right hemicolectomy.
    3. **Mid-transverse Colon:** Transverse colectomy or extended left or right hemicolectomy.
    4. **Splenic Flexure or Left Colon.** Left hemicolectomy.
    5. **Sigmoid Colon.** Sigmoid colectomy.
    6. **Upper or Middle Rectum.** Low anterior rectosigmoid resection with primary anastomosis.
    7. **Lower Rectum.** Abdominoperineal resection with permanent end colostomy, or local excision in selected cases.
- **D. Preoperative Bowel Preparation**
    1. Mechanical cleansing of the lumen, followed by decontamination with nonabsorbable oral antibiotics decreases the chance of infectious complications and allows for primary anastomosis.
    2. Partially obstructed patients should be prepped with caution because of the risk of perforation. Fully obstructed patients cannot be prepped and must have a temporary colostomy.
    3. Polyethylene glycol solution (CoLyte or GoLYTELY) is usually administered as 1 liter over 4 hours on the day before surgery. Nichols-Condon prep consists of 1 g neomycin sulfate and 1 g erythromycin base P.O. at 2:00, 3:00 and 11:00 pm the day before

operation. Cefotetan 1-2 gm IV 30 minutes before operation.
- **E.** Adjuvant chemotherapy based on 5-fluorouracil and levamisole for advanced colon lesions with the addition of pelvic radiation for advanced rectal tumors. Adjuvant therapy is reserved for locally advanced lesions (B2) or those with metastases to regional lymph nodes or distant organs (C1, C2, D).
- **F.** Staging workup (CT of chest, abdomen and pelvis) usually is done postoperatively since it is unnecessary for very early lesions, and it does not change operative management. Pathologic staging of the tumor is done postoperatively by histologic examination of the surgical specimen.

## IV. Staging of Colorectal Carcinoma

### A. Dukes' Classification
Stage A: Confined to the bowel wall.
Stage B: Extends through the bowel wall; lymph nodes negative.
Stage C: Metastatic to regional nodes.

### B. Astler-Coller Modification of Dukes' Classification (Most commonly used classification)
Stage A: Limited to mucosa and submucosa. Nodes negative.
Stage B1: Extends into but not through muscularis propria; nodes negative.
Stage B2: Extends through muscularis propria; nodes negative.
Stage C1: Same as B1, except nodes positive.
Stage C2: Same as B2, except nodes positive.

### C. TNM Classification (International standard)
TX: Tumor cannot be assessed.
T0: No tumor in specimen (prior polypectomy done).
Tis: Carcinoma in situ.
T1: Invades into submucosa.
T2: Invades into muscularis propria.
T3: Invades through muscularis propria.
T4: Invades adjacent organs or into free peritoneal cavity.
NX: Nodes cannot be assessed.
N0: No regional nodal metastasis.
N1: 1-3 nodes positive.
N2: More than 3 nodes positive.
N3: Central nodes positive.
MX: Presence of distant metastases cannot be assessed.
M0: No distant metastasis.
M1: Distant metastasis present.

## V. Management of Obstructing Carcinomas of the Left Colon

- **A.** Correct fluid deficits and electrolyte abnormalities. Nasogastric suction is useful, but it is not adequate to decompress the acutely obstructed colon.
- **B.** The Hartmann procedure is indicated for distal descending and sigmoid colon lesions. This procedure consists of resection of the obstructing cancer and formation of an end colostomy and blind rectal pouch. The colostomy can be taken down and anastomosed to the rectal pouch electively.
- **C.** Primary resection with temporary end colostomy and mucous fistula should be done for lesions of transverse and proximal descending colon. This procedure consists of resection of the obstructing cancer and creation of a functioning end colostomy and a defunctionalized distal limb with separate stomas. The colostomy can be taken down and continuity

      restored on an elective basis.
- D. An emergency decompressive loop colostomy can be considered for acutely ill patients. A hemicolectomy can be completed after four to six weeks.
- E. A primary anastomosis may be done in selected patients with a prepared bowel.

## VI. Management of Obstructing Carcinomas of the Ascending Colon
- A. Correct fluid deficits, and electrolyte abnormalities, and initiate nasogastric suction.
- B. A right hemicolectomy with primary anastomosis of the terminal ileum to the transverse colon can be performed on most patients. A temporary ileostomy is rarely needed.

**References:** See page 106.

# Mesenteric Ischemia and Infarction

## I. History
- A. **Acute.** Classic history of pain out of proportion to physical findings. Severe diffuse mid-abdominal pain (abrupt onset), bloody diarrhea, vomiting.
- B. **Chronic.** Colicky postprandial epigastric pain (mesenteric angina) often occurring 30-60 minutes after meals. Aversion to food, weight loss.
- C. History often includes peripheral vascular disease (claudication), coronary artery disease, atrial fibrillation, stroke, hyperlipidemia, diabetes.

## II. Physical Exam
- A. **General** Moderate to severe distress occurs in acute cases with cachexia.
- B. **Vitals.** Tachycardia, low-grade temperature elevation, orthostatic hypotension.
- C. **Heart.** Irregularly irregular rhythm (suggests emboli from atrial fibrillation).
- D. **Abdomen.** Diminished bowel sounds, abdominal bruits; often findings of tenderness or distention are minimal. Pulsatile supraumbilical mass suggests aortic aneurysm.
- E. **Rectal.** Occult or gross blood.
- F. **Extremities.** Diminished or absent pulses; bruits, loss of hair on legs, arterial ulcers, embolic gangrene of toes ("trash foot").
- G. Chronic mesenteric ischemia is associated with systemic vascular disease and weight loss.

## III. Laboratory Evaluation
- A. Electrolytes (prerenal azotemia, metabolic acidosis). CBC (leukocytosis).
- B. Abdominal series ("thumbprinting" suggests thickening of bowel wall; pneumatosis intestinalis portal vein gas).
- C. Mesenteric angiography confirms or excludes the diagnosis.

## IV. Differential Diagnosis. 
Peritonitis (secondary to acute appendicitis), acute cholecystitis, perforated viscus, peptic ulcer, gastroenteritis, pancreatitis, bowel obstruction, carcinoma, ruptured aortic aneurysm.

## V. Surgical Therapy of Mesenteric Infarction
- A. Acute mesenteric infarction is a surgical emergency. Main options include superior mesenteric artery thrombectomy, aortomesenteric bypass graft; superior mesenteric endarterectomy with patch angioplasty.
- B. A planned "second look" laparotomy may be used to confirm viability of bowel 24-48 hours after the initial revascularization.

# Intestinal Obstruction

I. **History**
   A. Crampy abdominal pain, vomiting, obstipation. History of previous laparotomy, hernia, colon cancer, gynecologic malignancy, cholelithiasis, chronic constipation, abdominal trauma; use of opiates, anticholinergics.
   B. Feculent emesis and distention suggests distal obstruction. Pain is often colicky at first; progressing to generalized, diffuse abdominal pain. Initially crampy or colicky pain with exacerbations at intervals of 5-10 minutes. Pain later becomes diffuse with fever. Localizes to periumbilical region in small bowel obstruction; localizes to lower abdomen in large bowel obstruction.
   C. Extremely severe pain suggests closed loop obstruction with intestinal ischemia.
   D. Immobilization, weight loss, recent pelvic or abdominal operation, electrolyte abnormalities, and some medications may predispose to adynamic small bowel ileus or colonic pseudo-obstruction (Ogilvie's syndrome).

II. **Physical Exam**
   A. **General:** Moderate to severe distress.
   B. **Vitals:** Tachycardia, orthostatic hypotension, fever.
   C. **Skin:** Cool, pale, clammy.
   D. **HEENT:** Fetid, foul breath.
   E. **Abdomen:** Healed laparotomy incisions, hernias (incisional, umbilical, epigastric, inguinal, femoral, obturator). Bowel sounds are initially increased with rushes and borborygmi; later, bowel sounds become decreased or silent. Distention, tympany to percussion. Diffuse rebound tenderness suggest peritonitis secondary to perforation.
   F. **Rectal:** The rectal vault may be empty or impacted with feces.

III. **Laboratory Evaluation**
   A. CBC (leukocytosis with left shift); electrolytes (hypokalemic, hypochloremic metabolic alkalosis from vomiting, or lactic acidosis from infarcted bowel).
   B. Amylase will be elevated in pancreatitis and bowel perforation.
   C. **Abdominal Films:** Dilated loops of small or large bowel with air/fluid levels and a "stairstep" appearance.
   D. Water-soluble contrast enema: Demonstrates large bowel obstruction or volvulus; the enema may resolve fecal impaction by inducing an osmotic diarrhea.

IV. **Differential Diagnosis of Intestinal Obstruction**
   A. **Causes of Small Bowel Obstruction:** Adhesions (previous laparotomy), hernias, inflammatory strictures, superior mesenteric artery syndrome, gallstone ileus, adynamic ileus, malnutrition, internal hernia.
   B. **Causes of Large Bowel Obstruction:** Colon cancer, sigmoid or cecal volvulus, diverticulitis, fecal impaction, adynamic ileus, pseudo-obstruction (Ogilvie's syndrome).

V. **Treatment of Intestinal Obstruction**
   A. Restore normal intravascular volume with fluid resuscitation. Place a Foley catheter and maintain urine output 0.5-1 mL/kg/hr. Correct hypokalemia and hypomagnesemia.

## 76 Intestinal Obstruction

- **B.** Initiate nasogastric suction (Levine tube to low intermittent suction). Replace the nasogastric output with an equal volume of 0.5 NS with 20-40 mEq/L potassium every 8 hours.
- **C. Small Bowel Obstruction**
  1. Nonoperative treatment with rehydration and nasogastric decompression is appropriate for partial obstructions thought to be due to adhesions. If such patients improve, continued nonoperative treatment is justified.
  2. Immediate operation is mandatory for obstructions due to strangulated hernias, and surgery should be strongly considered for all advanced or total obstructions.
- **D. Large Bowel Obstruction**
  1. A rapid workup should be performed to distinguish among impactions, pseudo-obstructions, and true obstructions of the colon. Manual disimpaction followed by hyperosmolar radiographic contrast enema is therapeutic for fecal impaction.
  2. Complete large bowel obstruction due to colon cancer, diverticulitis or volvulus require immediate laparotomy with resection of the obstructed segment. Primary anastomosis may be performed for right-sided lesions. Left sided colonic obstructions require a diverting end-colostomy and Hartmann pouch or mucous fistula.
  3. Colonoscopic decompression is standard treatment for Ogilvie's syndrome, and may permit nonoperative detorsion of a sigmoid volvulus.

# Acute Pancreatitis

## I. Diagnosis of Acute Pancreatitis

A. Pancreatitis usually presents as abdominal pain associated with elevated pancreatic enzymes. Pain is typically epigastric or in the left upper quadrant, and the pain is described as constant, dull, or boring; radiation of the pain to the mid-back and worsening in the supine position may occur.

B. Low-grade fever to 101°F is common. Higher temperature may indicate infectious complications. Acute pancreatitis may present with volume depletion, manifesting as hypotension or shock, because of vomiting, hemorrhage, or third spacing of fluid.

C. Patients may have a distended abdomen, and epigastric tenderness and localized rebound may be elicited.

D. Bleeding into the pancreatic bed may rarely manifest as ecchymoses of the flanks (Grey Turner's Sign) or as periumbilical bleeding (Cullen's sign).

## II. Etiology.
Identification of the etiology of an attack of pancreatitis is essential to prevent recurrences.

A. **Alcohol.** Alcoholic pancreatitis can develop after an alcohol binge.

B. **Gallstones**
   1. Ultrasonography visualizes gallstones in 75% of patients with "idiopathic" acute pancreatitis.
   2. **Conditions that Predispose to Biliary Stones.** Prolonged fasting (total parenteral nutrition, dieting), pregnancy.

C. **Hypertriglyceridemia** >1000 mg/dL may cause pancreatitis; lipid-reducing therapy will prevent recurrences.

D. **Abdominal Trauma.** Trauma such as an automobile accident can result in acute pancreatitis.

E. **Postoperative.** Pancreatitis may occur after upper abdominal, renal, or cardiovascular surgery.

F. **Hypercalcemia.** Pancreatitis has been reported with hypercalcemia.

G. **Pregnancy.** Pancreatitis is most likely during the third trimester and in the 6 weeks postpartum; it is usually related to alcohol or gallstones.

H. **Anatomic Causes.** Duodenal diverticula, choledochoceles, pancreatic or ampullary strictures, pancreas divisum, or tumors.

I. **Infections.** Viruses, parasites, and bacteria may cause pancreatitis.

J. **Vasculitis.** Pancreatitis may be a manifestation of vasculitis.

K. **Drugs.** Nonsteroidal anti-inflammatory drugs, erythromycin, thiazides, dideoxyinosine (ddI), pentamidine, sulfonamides, and 5-aminosalicylate.

L. **Other Causes.** Endoscopic retrograde cholangiopancreatography, hereditary pancreatitis, scorpion stings (Trinidad), organophosphate insecticides.

## III. Laboratory Evaluation

A. Elevated amylase is not pathognomonic for pancreatitis. Ruptured ectopic pregnancy, tubo-ovarian abscess, ovarian cysts, duodenal perforation, and mesenteric infarction may result in moderate hyperamylasemia. Clearance of amylase is reduced in renal failure, resulting in up to a threefold elevation.

B. In acute pancreatitis the amylase elevation is generally more pronounced than in other settings; values are usually at least 3 times normal. Mild hyperamylasemia may be seen in asymptomatic alcoholics and in acute cholecystitis or cholangitis.

## 78 Acute Pancreatitis

C. An elevated WBC count is common in pancreatitis.
D. **Isoamylase Determination:** Distinguishes pancreatic amylase from salivary amylase. Elevation of salivary isoamylase occurs with mumps, pneumonia, lung tumors, and breast or prostate cancers.
E. **Macroamylasemia**
  1. An elevation of serum amylase may result from low renal excretion of amylase, and is not an unusual finding in the normal population.
  2. Patients with macroamylasemia and pancreatitis may be diagnosed on the basis of an elevated serum lipase.
F. **Lipase** is more specific for pancreas than amylase.

IV. **Imaging Studies**
  A. **Radiographic Studies**
    1. Flat and upright films of the abdomen help exclude perforated viscus (free air under diaphragm).
    2. **Nonspecific Findings of Acute Pancreatitis:** Adynamic ileus or a sentinel loop (localized jejunal ileus). Pancreatic calcifications may be found with chronic pancreatitis.
  B. **Ultrasonography**
    1. Useful for evaluation of the biliary tract for gallstones.
    2. Acute pancreatitis is indicated by reduced pancreatic echogenicity, enlargement, or ductal dilation. The pancreas cannot be visualized in 40% because of overlying bowel gas.
  C. **Computed Tomography (CT) Scanning**
    1. Contrast-enhanced CT scans have a sensitivity of 90% and a specificity of 100% for the diagnosis of acute pancreatitis.
    2. **Indications for CT Scan:** Acute pancreatitis in patients who are seriously ill or if the diagnosis is uncertain.
  D. **Endoscopic Retrograde Cholangiopancreatography (ERCP):** Not routinely indicated during an attack of acute pancreatitis, but it may be useful in the following situations:
    1. Preoperative evaluation of traumatic pancreatitis.
    2. Suspected biliary pancreatitis with severe disease that is not improving and may need sphincterotomy and stone extraction.
    3. In patients older than 40 years with no identifiable cause, ERCP is indicated once the attack of pancreatitis has subsided to determine the etiology.

V. **Assessment of Prognosis**
  A. **Ranson's Criteria**
    1. Used to assess prognosis early in the course of acute pancreatitis.
    2. Overall, mortality from acute pancreatitis is approximately 1% in patients with less than 3 signs, 15% with 3 or 4 signs, 40% with 5 or 6 signs, and 100% with 7 or more signs.

## Ranson's Criteria for Alcoholic Pancreatitis

| At Admission: | During Initial 48 Hours: |
|---|---|
| 1. Age over 55 years | 1. Hematocrit drop >10% points |
| 2. WBC >16,000/mm$^3$ | 2. BUN rise >5 mg/dL |
| 3. Blood glucose >200 mg/dL (in a nondiabetic) | 3. Arterial PO2 <60 mm Hg |
| 4. Serum LDH >350 IU/L | 4. Base deficit >4 mEq/L |
| 5. AST >250 U/L | 5. Serum calcium <8.0 mg/dL |
| | 6. Estimated fluid sequestration >6 L |

## Ranson's Criteria for Nonalcoholic Pancreatitis

**Admission**
1. Age over 70 years
2. WBC >18,000/mm³
3. Blood glucose >220 mg/dL (in a nondiabetic)
4. Serum LDH >400 IU/L
5. AST >250 U/L

**Initial 48 hours**
1. Hematocrit drop >10% points
2. BUN rise >2 mg/dL
3. Base deficit >5 mEq/L
4. Serum calcium <8.0 mg/dL
5. Estimated fluid sequestration >4 L

## VI. Complications of Pancreatitis
A. **Pseudocyst** is a pancreatic fluid collection that may regress, or it may progress to a mature pseudocyst.
B. **Necrotizing pancreatitis** occurs after infection of the necrotic pancreatic tissue, often within 6 days after the episode begins.
C. **Shock, adult respiratory distress syndrome** (ARDS), renal failure, and gastrointestinal bleeding are occasional complications.

## VII. Medical Management of Pancreatitis
A. **Supportive Medical Care for Local and Systemic Complications.** The majority of patients (>80%) have rapid resolution of the inflammatory process and a noncomplicated course.
B. **Replace Intravascular Volume.** Ringer's lactate, normal saline or colloids (albumin) are administer to restore hemodynamic stability and to maintain a urine output of 0.5-1 cc/kg/h. Monitor central venous pressure and replace calcium and magnesium deficits.
C. **Pancreatic Rest.** Oral feeding is withheld until nausea, vomiting, and abdominal pain have subsided. Total parenteral nutrition is usually necessary. After acute symptoms have resolved, feeding may be started, with gradual progression from liquids to a regular diet.
D. **Nasogastric Suction** is used if severe nausea, vomiting, or ileus is present.
E. **Antibiotics.** Prophylactic antibiotics are used with a temperature >101.5°F, cholangitis, or severe pancreatitis. Cefoxitin (Mefoxin) 1-2 gm IV q6h **OR**
Cefotetan (Cefotan) 1-2 gm IV q12h.
F. **Analgesics.** Meperidine (Demerol) should be used because morphine may cause spasm of the sphincter of Oddi.
G. **Medical Management**
  1. Somatostatin 250 mcg IV bolus, followed by 100 mcg/h x 48 hours **OR**
  2. Octreotide (Sandostatin) 100-200 mcg SC three times per day.
  3. Ranitidine (Zantac) 50 mg IV q8h **OR**
  4. Cimetidine (Tagamet) 300 mg IV q8h.
  5. Insulin may be needed if there is severe hyperglycemia.
  6. Alcohol withdrawal prophylaxis may be required with chlordiazepoxide 50-100 mg IV/IM q6h round the clock x 3 days, thiamine 100 mg IM/IV qd x 3d; folic acid 1 mg IM/IV qd x 3d; multivitamin qd.

## VIII. Surgical Management of Pancreatitis
A. **Surgical Management** is indicated to exclude other intra-abdominal processes, or if abscess, infection, necrotizing pancreatitis, or pseudocyst.
B. Operative management should be guided by CT imaging.
C. A cholecystectomy is indicated for biliary pancreatitis. The procedure is usually performed early, usually on hospital day 3 or 4 when amylase has

returned to normal. Surgery may be performed during the acute attack if deterioration occurs. Endoscopic sphincterotomy is useful to remove obstructing stones.
   D. Severe necrotizing pancreatitis requires necrosectomy to remove necrotic pancreatic tissue and septic material. This is followed by local lavage and placement of drains.
IX. **Pancreatic Pseudocyst**
   A. Clinical signs of pseudocyst include continuing abdominal pain, vomiting, nausea, epigastric tenderness, abdominal mass, and hyperamylasemia. CT and ultrasound are diagnostic.
   B. **Pseudocyst Management**
      1. Pseudocysts are managed expectantly for 6-8 weeks until a mature cyst wall develops.
      2. Pseudocysts that are less than 5 cm in diameter usually resolve spontaneously.
      3. After a mature cyst wall has developed, internal drainage by cystogastrostomy, cystojejunostomy, or cystoduodenostomy is completed. A malignant pseudocyst should be excluded by biopsy of cyst wall.
      4. Percutaneous, CT guided drainage may be considered after thickening of cyst wall has occurred.

**References:** See page 106.

# Cholecystitis and Cholelithiasis

I. **Clinical Evaluation**
   A. **History:** Acute cholecystitis is characterized by biliary colic, constant, right upper quadrant pain, occurring 30-90 minutes after meals, lasting several hours. The pain may extend to the epigastrium and radiate to back or right scapula. Pain has an abrupt onset with gradual relief. Pain is low grade fever 99-101°F. Nausea, vomiting, anorexia.
   B. Fatty food intolerance, dark urine, clay colored stools; bloating, jaundice, flatulence, obesity. Asian patients have an increased incidence of pigment stones.
   C. History of gallstones, alcohol. History of fasting; high calorie diets, estrogen, diabetes.
   D. Charcot's triad: right upper quadrant pain, jaundice, fever and chills, indicates ascending cholangitis.
II. **Physical Exam**
   A. **Vital Signs.** P (mild tachycardia), T (low-grade fever), R (shallow respirations), BP (hypotension).
   B. **Abdomen.** Epigastric or right upper quadrant tenderness, Murphy's sign (increased tenderness and inspiratory arrest during deep palpation of RUQ); guarding; rigidity, rebound.
III. **Laboratory Evaluation**
   A. Moderate leukocytosis; mild elevation of bilirubin, increased alkaline phosphatase, AST, amylase. (If amylase is greater than 1000 U, consider biliary pancreatitis).
   B. **Radionuclide scan (HIDA).** Positive if gallbladder does not visualize within 4 hours and radioisotope is visible in the common bile duct. Useful if bilirubin is less than 9 mg %, but may give a false positive if patient has

not eaten for more than 48 hours.
- **C.** Ultrasound of right upper quadrant shows dilation and gallstones; bile duct wall thickening, liver abscess, gas in biliary tree.
- **D. Plain Abdominal X-ray.** Enlarged gallbladder shadow; calcifications in gallbladder; air in gallbladder wall (emphysematous cholecystitis); imprint of distended gallbladder on duodenum.

## IV. Differential Diagnosis.
Cholecystitis, cholangitis, peptic ulcer, pancreatitis, appendicitis, gastroesophageal reflux disease, hepatitis, nephrolithiasis, hepatic metastases, gonococcal perihepatitis, pneumonia, angina.

## V. Complications.
Perforated gallbladder, cholangitis, cholecystenteric fistula, gallstone ileus (stone passes into intestinal lumen via a fistula, and causes obstruction).

## VI. Treatment
- **A.** Remove the inflamed gallbladder during the acute stage (open or laparoscopic cholecystectomy).
- **B.** Initially conservative, nonoperative measures (antibiotics, analgesics); followed later by elective cholecystectomy in a few weeks or months, after acute inflammation has resolved.
- **C. Conservative Therapy**
    1. Antibiotics, IV fluids, electrolyte replacement. Operative drainage, should be considered for toxic patients for decompression of biliary tree.
    2. **IV Fluids:** Give IV crystalloids to restore intravascular volume. NG tube (10-18 F) at low constant suction (if nausea or vomiting); no oral intake.
    3. **Special Medications**
        a. Gentamicin, 1.5-2 mg/kg, then 2-5 mg/kg/d IV **AND**
        b. Metronidazole (Flagyl) 1.0 gm (15 mg/kg) over 1h, then 500 mg (7.5 mg/kg) IV q6h **OR**
        c. Ticarcillin/Clavulanate (Timentin) 3.1 g IV q4-6h **OR**
        d. Piperacillin/tazobactam (Zosyn) 4.5 gm IV q6h.
    4. **Symptomatic Medications**
        a. Meperidine (Demerol) 50-100 mg IM q4-6h prn pain.

# Management of the Cholecystectomy Patient

## I. Evaluation Before Early Cholecystectomy
- **A.** Confirm diagnosis with ultrasound and HIDA scan. Administer parenteral antibiotics and volume resuscitation.
    1. E. coli is the most common pathogen after cholecystectomy. With common duct obstruction, other pathogens, including Klebsiella spp, enterococcus, Clostridia spp, also are significant.
    2. Recommended prophylaxis consists of cefazolin (however, enterococcus coverage should be added in the "septic-appearing patient".
- **B.** Do not delay surgery in extremely ill patients with a palpable gallbladder or if complications develop such as emphysematous cholecystitis.
- **C.** Cholecystectomy may be performed in good risk patients presenting <72 hours after onset of symptoms.
- **D.** If the patient improves, early nonoperative conservative treatment may be considered with elective cholecystectomy scheduled at a later date. If the

## Laparoscopic Cholecystectomy Procedure

I. **Advantages of Laparoscopic Surgery:** Usually less postoperative; pain; reduced recovery time; several small puncture wounds instead of a large surgical incision; early return to work.

II. **Procedure**
   A. Insert a Hasson cannula through infraumbilical incision, and distend the peritoneal cavity with gas.
   B. The gallbladder is removed by inserting cannulae, special probes and instruments into abdominal cavity under video visualization.
   C. An intraoperative cholangiogram may be performed during laparoscopy.

III. **Contraindications to Laparoscopic Cholecystectomy:** Adhesions, extreme gallbladder scarring, severe acute inflammation, bleeding, and other technically difficult situations.

## Open Cholecystectomy Procedure

A. Prior to surgery place a nasogastric tube to decompress the stomach. The most commonly used incision is the Kocher's right subcostal.

B. Place incision 4 cm below and parallel to the costal margin, and extend it from the midline to the anterior axillary line. Open the anterior rectus sheath with a knife in the line of the incision. Divide the rectus muscle, and open the peritoneum between forceps.

C. Systematically explore the peritoneal cavity and note the appearance of the hiatus, stomach, duodenum, liver, pancreas, intestines, and kidneys. Palpate the gallbladder from the ampulla towards the fundus; then palpate the common duct, noting any dilation or foreign bodies. Carefully palpate colon for neoplasms.

D. Grasp the gallbladder with a Rochester-Pean or Pennington clamp near the fundus. Hold forceps in one hand, and introduce the right hand over the right lobe of the liver, permitting the liver to descend. Divide any adhesions to the omentum, colon or duodenum, and place a pack over these structures, then retract the structures inferiorly with a broad-bladed Deaver's retractor.

E. Inspect the anatomy of the biliary tree by carefully dividing the peritoneum covering the anterior aspect of the cystic duct, and continue dissecting into the anterior layer of the lesser omentum overlying the common bile duct. Bluntly dissect with a blunt dissector (Kitner), exposing Charcot's triangle bounded by the cystic duct, common bile duct and inferior border of the liver. The cystic artery should be seen in this triangle. Carefully observe the arrangement of the duct system and arterial supply. Do not divide any structure until the anatomy has been identified, including the cystic duct, common bile duct and porta hepatitis structures.

F. Pass a ligature around the cystic duct with a right-angle clamp, and make a loose knot near the common duct. Partially divide the cystic duct below the infundibulum, and place a small polyethylene catheter, attached to a syringe filled with saline, into the cystic duct for 1-2 cm. Tighten the

## Laparoscopic Cholecystectomy Procedure

ligature holding the catheter in position.

G. Attach a second syringe containing contrast material to the catheter, and remove all instruments. Place a sterile sheet, and slowly inject 15 cc of diluted dye into the common duct. Evaluate an operative cholangiogram to detect stones and evaluate the duct system. Make an X-ray exposure, then reposition table and make an exposure. Uncover the wound and proceed while the X-rays are processed.

H. Palpate the lower end of common bile duct and pancreas. Insert the index finger of the left hand into the foramen of Winslow. Allow the index finger to lie posterior to the second part of the duodenum and the head of the pancreas, and examine the pancreas for abnormal thickening due to inflammation, or stony hardness due to tumor. Palpate the ampulla, checking for stones or tumor. Hold the forceps on the gallbladder in the left hand to produce tension, and clear the cystic artery of soft tissue with a pledget held in forceps. Follow the artery to the gallbladder, and clamp it with a right angle clamp. Divide and ligate the artery close to the edge of the gallbladder, using clips or 000 silk.

I. Reaffirm the junction of the cystic duct with the common bile, then completely divide the exposed cystic duct, leaving a stump of at least 5 mm.

J. Hold the two forceps on the gallbladder in the left hand to put tension on the tissues between the gall bladder and the liver. Incise the peritoneum anteriorly over the gallbladder with a scalpel. Elevate the peritoneum from the gallbladder, and separate the gallbladder gently with sharp and blunt dissection. Tissue strands containing vessels should be cauterized before division.

K. Inspect the gallbladder bed for bleeding which may be cauterized or ligated. Control any persistent oozing from the bed with a small pack of hemostatic gauze.

L. Irrigate the site with saline. Routine drainage is unnecessary. However, if there is excessive fluids, place a soft rubber Penrose drain or closed suction drain in the area of the dissection, and bring it out through a separate stab wound in the right upper quadrant if desired. Inspect the operative field, including the ligatures on the arteries and the cystic duct. Grasp the peritoneum with a series of Kocher's forceps in continuity with the posterior rectus sheath, and approximate it with continuous nonabsorbable suture.

M. Irrigate the wound with saline and ligate any bleeding vessels. Approximate the rectus fascia and fascia of the oblique muscles with interrupted, nonabsorbable sutures. Irrigate the subcutaneous space with saline and close skin with staples, or absorbable subcuticular sutures. Secure the drain with a suture, and identify it with a safety pin. Cover the wound with a dressing.

**84 Open Cholecystectomy Procedure**

# Breast Cancer

John A. Butler, M.D.

## Evaluation of Breast Masses

### I. Recommended Intervals for Breast Cancer Screening Studies

|  | Age <40 yr | 40-49 yr | 50-75 yr |
|---|---|---|---|
| **Breast Self-Examination** | Monthly by age 30 | Monthly | Monthly |
| **Professional Breast Examination** | Every 3 yr, ages 20-39 | Annually | Annually |
| **Mammography High-risk Patient** | Baseline at 35-39 yr | Annually | Annually |
| **Low-risk Patient** |  | Baseline at 40, then optional | Annually |

### II. Differential Diagnosis of Breast Masses
  A. **<30 Years Old.** The common causes are fibroadenoma, papillomatosis, abscess (especially if lactating), and fat necrosis.
  B. **30-50 Years Old.** Common causes include fibrocystic mastopathy, cancer, fatty lobule, or cystosarcoma phylloides.
  C. **Older than 50.** Cancer is the primary diagnosis, followed by fibrocystic mastopathy, fat necrosis, and cyst.

### III. Clinical Evaluation of Breast Masses
  A. The history should assess how long the mass has been present, associated pain (especially if cyclical), any change in size, and the color of any nipple discharge.
  B. Determine results of, and time since, the last clinical breast examination and the last mammogram.
  C. **Risk Factors.** A risk assessment is undertaken for breast cancer risk factors, including patient age over 50 years, past personal history of breast cancer, history of hyperplasia on previous breast biopsies, and family history of breast cancer in a first-degree relatives (mother, sister, daughter). 80% of women with breast cancer have no risk factors other than being women and over 50 years old.
  D. **Physical Examination**
   1. The patient then should sit up with arms first at her side and then behind her head, this facilitates examination of the breast contours and allows visualization of nipple inversion or tethering.
   2. Examine for dimpling, asymmetry, lumps, thickened areas, or shape or contour. Compress nipples to identify any discharge and palpate both axillae. Assess masses for multiple components, mobility, and

cystic or solid qualities. A drawing should be made of any irregularities or masses.
3. The patient is examined in the supine position with her arms up and behind her head, this flattens the breast tissue and compresses it for examination.
4. Very discrete, smooth nodules are more likely to be benign; tenderness is associated with benignity.

## IV. Triple Test Diagnosis of Breast Masses

A. In the triple test, a palpable breast nodule is assessed by physical exam, mammography, and aspiration biopsy.
B. Each test taken individually has a significant false negative rate. However, taken together, the tests have a false negative rate equal to a surgical biopsy. The false negative rate for the triple test is 0.4%, compared with the 0.5-1% rate for surgical diagnosis.
C. If the clinical exam, mammography, and fine-needle aspiration biopsy are benign, open biopsy is usually not necessary. A benign breast nodule by triple test can be managed by conservative follow-up, with breast self examination and professional examinations over 2-3 years.
D. Any mass that is either clinically or mammographically suspicious for cancer generally requires excisional biopsy, even if the fine needle aspiration biopsy is benign.
E. Mammography is usually not clinically appropriate for patients under 35 years old. For this group, the double test of physical examination and cytologic examination is sufficient.
F. An ultrasound of the breast may sometimes be obtained to determine if the mass is cystic or solid. If the lesion is cystic, no further management is necessary, or the fluid can be removed and the cyst collapsed by needle aspiration. If the mass is solid, fine needle aspiration biopsy is recommended.
G. **Fine-Needle Aspiration Biopsy (FNAB)**
   1. The skin is prepped with alcohol and the lesion is immobilized by the nonoperating hand. A 10 mL syringe with a 18 to 22 gauge needle is introduced in to the central portion of the mass at a 90° angle. When the needle enters the mass, suction is applied by retracting the plunger, and the needle is advanced. The needle is directed into different areas of the mass while maintaining suction on the syringe.
   2. Suction is slowly released before the needle is withdrawn from the mass. The contents of the needle is placed onto glass slides for pathologic examination.
H. **Cyst Aspiration.** If the physical characteristics (or ultrasound) support the diagnosis of a cyst, needle aspiration may be done.
   1. Using the same technique as for FNAB, the cyst fluid is evacuated.
   2. Successful aspiration of a simple cyst will yield nonbloody fluid followed by complete resolution of the mass. Watery fluid may be discarded. However, cyst fluid that is bloody or unusually tenacious, should be examined cytologically.
   3. If the lesion is found to be solid or if no fluid is obtained, the needle is used to aspirate tissue as in a FNAB.
   4. A residual mass after aspiration or presence of a bloody aspirate requires open biopsy. Before the referral, a mammogram should be obtained for any patient over age 35 who has not had a mammogram within the preceding 6 months.

## V. Evaluation of Breast Lesions Detected by Screening Mammography

A. For any lesions identified as demonstrating micro-calcifications that suggest cancer, referral for open biopsy is recommended.
B. Any lesions identified as having architectural distortion or interval growth when compared with a previous mammogram, should be referred for open biopsy.

**References:** See page 106.

# Excisional Breast Biopsy Technique

A. When mammography demonstrates a lesion suggestive of malignancy, the patient should have a mammogram on the morning of the operation and wire probes placed in the lesion for localization.
B. Infiltrate the skin and underlying tissues with 1% lidocaine with epinephrine. For lesions located within 5 cm of the nipple, a periareolar incision may be used of no more than half the areola circumference, or use a curved incision located over the mass and parallel to the areola.
C. Incise the skin and subcutaneous fat, then palpate the lesion and excise the mass. Send the specimen with the wire probes in place, for radiography to ensure that the abnormality has been fully exercised.
D. Close the wound with a 4-0 chromic catgut suture for the subcutaneous tissues, and 4-0 subcuticular Dexon for the skin.

# Urology

C. Garo Gholdoian, M.D.
David A. Chamberlin, M.D.

## Prostate Cancer

The average age at diagnosis of prostate cancer is 73 years. The age-adjusted death rate from prostate cancer has not changed appreciably in 35 years.

**I. Clinical Evaluation**
   A. The prevalence of prostate cancer is 30% in men over the age of 50. One in six men will be diagnosed with prostate cancer during their lifetimes.
   B. Some patients with prostate cancer may have obstructive urinary symptoms similar to benign prostatic hypertrophy; some patients may have weight loss and bone pain. Most patients have no symptoms, only an elevated prostate specific antigen found on routine screening.
   C. **Physical Exam:** Digital rectal exam is used to assess the nodule for extension beyond prostate edge, firmness, fixation, or induration.
   D. **Prostate Specific Antigen (PSA)**
      1. PSA is a glycoprotein produced by both benign and malignant prostatic epithelium.
      2. Each gram of prostate tissue increases serum PSA by about 0.3 ng/mL, but each gram of prostate cancer increases serum PSA by about 3.5 ng/mL.
      3. **PSA screening** improves detection of prostate cancer at an earlier stage. However, an improvement in survival has not yet been proven.

**Normal Prostate Specific Antigen Levels (Age Adjusted)**

| Age (years) | Normal Level (ng/mL) |
|---|---|
| 40-50 | <2.5 |
| 51-60 | <3.5 |
| 61-70 | <4.5 |
| >70 | <6.5 |

(Oesterling et al)

   4. A normal PSA does not rule out prostate cancer at any stage. However, a level above 10 ng/mL (and especially above 20 ng/mL) almost certainly reflects malignancy. Serial PSA levels that are increasing, even if still <10 ng/mL, probably indicate tumor.
   5. A PSA > 4.0 ng/mL detects 46% of subsequently diagnosed prostate cancers, with a specificity of 91%.
   6. PSA levels between 2 and 3 ng/mL were associated with a 5-fold

increased risk of developing prostate cancer.
7. There is no effect of rectal exam on PSA when the level is low. However, there are substantial increases when the initial PSA is >10 ng/mL. Instrumentation and prostatic massage cause greater increases in PSA.

### E. Transrectal Ultrasonography
1. Transrectal ultrasound is more sensitive than digital rectal exam, but still misses about 30% of known cancers.
2. The main indication of ultrasound is to guide transrectal prostate biopsy.

## II. Urological Evaluation of Suspected Prostate Cancer
A. The prostate nodule is evaluated by transrectal ultrasound and prostate needle biopsies. If no transrectal ultrasound lesion is identified, then random sextet biopsies should be performed.
B. **Indications for Biopsy:** (1) Abnormal digital rectal exam (discrete, firm nodule), (2) Elevated prostate-specific antigen (regardless of digital rectal exam).
C. **Metastatic Evaluation.** SMA 18, chest x-ray, intravenous pyelogram or ultrasound (optional), and bone scan.

## III. Staging of Prostate Cancer

### Tumor Node Metastases Classification (TNM)

| Tumor stage | TNM |
|---|---|
| **Incidental finding (TURP)** | |
| ≤3 microscopic foci (≤5%) | T1a |
| >3 microscopic loci (>5%) | T1b |
| Increased PSA | T1c |
| **Clinical tumor, limited to prostate** | |
| ≤1.5 cm | T2a |
| >1.5 cm or >1 lobe | T2b |
| **Tumor beyond prostate** | |
| Not in seminal vesicles | T3 |
| Seminal vesicles | T3 |
| Fixed to pelvis, or invades locally | T4 |
| **Metastatic disease** | |
| Lymph nodes | N |
| Distant | M |

### Histopathologic Grade (Gleason Score)

| | |
|---|---|
| Well-differentiated, slight anaplasia | (1-4) |
| Moderate well-differentiated, moderate anaplasia | (5-7) |
| Poorly differentiated, marked anaplasia | (8-10) |

## Combining grade and TNM yields final stage

| Stage A₁ |           | T1a or T2a    | and | Gleason ≤4 |
|----------|-----------|---------------|-----|------------|
| A₂       | Stage I   | T1a or T2a    |     |            |
| B        | Stage II  | T1b, T2b      | and | Any        |
| C        | Stage III | T3            | and | Any        |
| D        | Stage IV  | T4 or N or M  | and | Any        |

### IV. Therapy of Early Stage Prostate Cancer
A. Stage 0 disease can be followed
B. Stage I and II disease are best managed surgically with radical prostatectomy (with radiation therapy another option). Radical prostatectomy consists of removal of the prostate and seminal vesicles, and a staging pelvic lymph node dissection.
C. Stage III disease is managed with radiotherapy or surgery.
D. Stage IV disease is managed with endocrine manipulation.
E. There is no firm evidence that any of these therapies is better than any other: therefore, "watchful waiting" is also a legitimate option in selected patients.
F. **Endocrine Therapy of Advanced Prostate Carcinoma**
   1. Treatment of advanced malignancy (Stage IV) involves surgical or medical castration.
   2. Total blockade (eg, leuprolide plus flutamide) is slightly better than leuprolide alone.
   3. Orchiectomy is an outpatient procedure that is the safest and least expensive option. There is no higher incidence of impotence with orchiectomy than with medical castration therapies.

**References:** See page 106.

# Renal Colic

Approximately 5% of the U.S. population will pass a urinary tract stone during their lifetime.

### I. Pathophysiology
A. Calcium-containing stones are the most common (70%).
B. Magnesium-ammonium-phosphate stones, also known as struvite stones, are almost always associated with urinary tract infection by urea-splitting bacteria such as Proteus mirabilis. These are generally responsible for large staghorn calculi stones.
C. Uric acid stones are less common and are radiolucent, making diagnosis by plain films alone difficult.
D. Cystine stones are rare and associated with cystinuria, a rare autosomal recessive hereditary disorder.

### II. Clinical Evaluation
A. Renal colic is characterized as severe colicky pain that is intermittent,

# Renal Colic

usually in the flank or lower abdomen. Patients usually can not find a "comfortable position," and the pain often radiates to the testes or groin. A history of previous stones, poor fluid intake, urinary tract infections, or hematuria is common.

    B. Obstruction located at the ureteropelvic junction causes pure flank pain, while upper ureteral obstruction causes flank pain that radiates to the groin. Midureteral stones cause lower abdominal pain and may mimic appendicitis or diverticulitis, but without localized point tenderness or guarding. Lower ureteral stones may cause irritative voiding symptoms and scrotal or labial pain.

    C. Patients with nephrolithiasis generally complain of nausea and vomiting. They commonly have gross or microscopic hematuria; fever and increased white blood cell count are also possible.

    D. Prior episodes of renal colic or a family history of renal stones is often reported.

    E. **Physical Examination**
1. Generally the patient is agitated, diaphoretic, and unable to find a comfortable position.
2. Hypertension and tachycardia are also common.
3. Costovertebral angle tenderness is the classic physical finding; however, minimal abdominal tenderness without guarding, rebound, or rigidity may be present. Right or left lower quadrant tenderness or an enlarged kidney may sometimes be noted.

III. **Differential Diagnosis.** Appendicitis, salpingitis, diverticulitis, pyelonephritis, ovarian torsion, prostatitis, ectopic pregnancy, bowel obstruction, carcinoma.

IV. **Laboratory Evaluation**

    A. A urinalysis with microscopic, serum chemistries, BUN, creatinine, complete blood count, and urine culture should be obtained. An elevated white blood cell count may occur, and when it is associated with fever, its presence usually indicates an associated infection. A significant number of white cells in the urine also suggests infection.

    B. A plain abdominal film may demonstrate a calcification along the course of the urinary tract, as 90% of all calculi are radiopaque. These films, however, are highly inaccurate, since calcifications may either be missed because of overlying bowel gas, or calcifications may be related to processes outside the urinary tract.

    C. **Intravenous Pyelogram**
1. IVP is considered the gold standard, and it allows rapid assessment of the degree of obstruction, location of the stone and any renal function impairment.
2. In cases of acute ureteral obstruction, the classic findings are a dense nephrogram with a delay in excretion of contrast. Visualization of the whole ureter above the stone (columnization) is sometimes demonstrated.

    D. **Ultrasound** has a limited role in the evaluation of acute renal colic, but it may be useful in patients with renal failure or an intravenous contrast allergy.

V. **Management of Renal Calculi**

    A. Most renal calculi will pass spontaneously, and only expectant management with hydration and analgesia is necessary.

    B. Obstruction associated with fever indicates urinary tract infection, and it requires prompt drainage with either a ureteral stent or percutaneous nephrostomy to prevent sepsis.

**C. Indications for Admission**
1. High fever, uncontrollable pain
2. Intractable nausea and vomiting with an inability to tolerate oral fluids
3. Solitary kidney

**D. Inpatient Management**
1. Vigorous intravenous hydration and intravenous antibiotics are important when infection is suspected.
2. Parenteral narcotics are often necessary.
3. Ketorolac (Toradol), an IM nonsteroidal drug, is effective and provides a good alternative to narcotics.
4. Strain all urine in an attempt to retrieve spontaneously passed stones for X-ray crystallography analysis.

**E.** Stones measuring 5 to 10 mm have a decreased likelihood of passage, and early elective intervention should be considered

**F.** Extracorporeal shock-wave lithotripsy (ESWL) is the most common procedure for small renal or ureteral stones. 80% of patients become stone-free after one treatment.

**G.** Ureteroscopy with laser, ultrasound or electrohydraulic lithotripsy may be used as well. Open surgical stone removal is rarely necessary.

**H. Outpatient Management**
1. Most patients with renal colic do not require admission.
2. Most stones measuring less than 4 mm will pass spontaneously (90-95%), and approximately 80% of these will pass within 4 weeks.
3. Patients should increase intake of oral fluids, take narcotic pain medication, and strain all urine.
4. Close follow-up is necessary and plain abdominal films may be used to assess movement of the stone.

**I. Follow up Care**
1. After the stone has passed, a metabolic evaluation is important because 70% of patients will have a repeat stones if not diagnosed.
2. Evaluation may include chemistry screening, calcium, uric acid, phosphorous, UA with micro, urine C&S, urine cystine (nitroprusside test), 24 hour urine collection for uric acid, calcium, creatinine. If increased serum calcium, check PTH level.

**References:** See page 106.

# Urologic Emergencies

**I. Acute Urinary Retention**
  **A.** Acute urinary retention is characterized by a sudden inability to void. It often presents with suprapubic pain and severe urgency. There is usually a history of preexisting obstructive voiding symptoms related to bladder outlet obstruction or poor detrusor function.
  **B. Complications of Acute Urinary Retention**
  1. Postobstructive diuresis
  2. Bladder mucosal hemorrhage
  3. Hypotension
  4. Sepsis
  5. Renal failure

## Urologic Emergencies

6. Autonomic bladder hyporeflexia

C. **Benign prostatic hyperplasia** is the most common cause of acute urinary retention in men over the age of 50.
   1. Patients present with progressively worsening voiding difficulties, resulting in bladder overdistention and subsequent urinary retention.
   2. Prostate size on digital rectal examination has no bearing on the degree of outlet obstruction because minimal enlargement of the prostate can cause significant obstruction in some patients.

D. **Prostate cancer** accounts for 25% of patients with acute urinary retention. 10% of patients with prostate cancer initially present with bladder outlet obstruction.

E. **Additional Causes of Acute Urinary Retention:** Urethral strictures, bladder neck contractures, bladder stones, and acute bacterial prostatitis.

F. **Poor bladder function** can cause acute urinary retention. Common causes of poor bladder function include prolonged obstruction, diabetes mellitus, neurologic disorders (spinal cord injury, herniated vertebral disk, dementia), and medications.

G. **Urinary retention after surgery** sometimes temporarily develops in elderly men. There is usually preexisting bladder dysfunction or outlet obstruction that predisposes the patient to urinary retention.

H. **Anticholinergic medications** (antihistamines, antidiarrheals, antispasmodics, tricyclic antidepressants) can suppress bladder function. Sympathomimetic drugs (decongestants and diet pills) that cause contraction of the smooth muscle in the bladder neck can precipitate an increase in outlet resistance.

I. **Clinical Evaluation of Acute Urinary Retention**
   1. Retention is characterized by an inability to void and suprapubic discomfort. A progressive history of difficulty voiding and irritative voiding symptoms, such as frequency, nocturia, or urgency is often noted.
   2. Some patients are incontinent as a result of extreme overdistention of the bladder.
   3. A past history of gonorrhea or trauma, that may have caused a stricture, should be sought, as well as the presence of underlying diseases and medications.
   4. Palpate for a distended bladder and assess size and consistency of the prostate. Tenderness of the prostate on rectal examination suggests acute prostatitis; a diffusely hard or nodular prostate indicates carcinoma.
   5. The penis should be examined to rule out phimosis, paraphimosis, or meatal stenosis.
   6. A neurologic exam should be completed including anal sphincter reflex and perineal sensation.
   7. **Laboratory Evaluation:** Serum electrolytes, blood urea nitrogen (BUN), creatinine, urinalysis, and culture.

J. **Management of Acute Urinary Retention**
   1. Prompt drainage of the entire bladder contents with a Foley catheter is essential. Adequate volume replacement is necessary to prevent hypotension.
   2. Lubrication with 2% lidocaine jelly (injected directly into the urethra with a syringe) will facilitate insertion of a urethral catheter.
   3. Medium-sized catheters (#18 to #22 French) should be used because

they tend to be stiffer and easier to insert than smaller ones, which can coil within the urethra.
4. In patients with large prostates, coude catheters, which have a curved tip, may be helpful. The curve of the coude catheter should be directed superiorly. Other methods of drainage include urethral sounds, filiforms with followers, and percutaneous suprapubic tubes.
5. Admission to the hospital is not required for most patients with acute urinary retention unless other associated factors, such as infection or renal failure, are present. Most patients can be managed with a Foley catheter and discharged home with oral antibiotics and a leg urine bag.

### K. Complications of Acute Urinary Retention
1. Postobstructive diuresis can occur; therefore, fluid and electrolyte balance should be monitored closely.
2. If significant post-drainage hemorrhage occurs, continuous bladder irrigation should be initiated.
3. Hypotension may result from either hypovolemia or a vasovagal reaction. However, it can be prevented by adequate volume replacement. Slow decompression of the bladder is not recommended.
4. Other complications of urinary retention include sepsis and renal failure due to longstanding obstruction.

## II. Testicular Torsion
A. Testicular torsion is an emergency, and any delay in treatment may result in testicular loss. A four- to six-hour delay may damage normal testicular function.
B. Torsion can occur at any age; however, it is most common in adolescents, peaking at the age of 15 to 16 years.
C. Testicular torsion presents with sudden onset of pain and swelling in one testicle, occasionally associated with minor trauma. There is frequently nausea, vomiting, and lower abdominal or flank pain. There may be a history of previous similar episodes with spontaneous resolution.
D. A urinalysis is essential in differentiating testicular torsion from epididymitis; however, a negative urinalysis does not rule out epididymitis, since it may be of the sterile variant.

### E. Differential Diagnosis of Testicular Torsion
1. Epididymitis due to Neisseria gonorrhoeae and Chlamydia trachomatis is much more common than torsion in adult men.
2. Torsion of an appendix testis or appendix epididymis may also mimic testicular torsion. Torsion of the appendix testis may manifest as a tender, pea-sized nodule at the upper pole of the testicle with a small blue-black dot seen through the scrotal skin (the blue dot sign); management is conservative. If there is diagnostic uncertainty, surgical exploration is required.
3. Other less common conditions that may present similarly to torsion include acute hemorrhage into a testicular neoplasm, orchitis, testicular abscess, incarcerated hernia, and testicular rupture.

### F. Physical Examination
1. Testicular torsion usually presents with severe unilateral testicular pain with an acute onset. The pain is associated with an extremely tender testicle with a transverse lie or an anterior epididymis that lies high in the scrotum.

2. The testis is high in the scrotum (Brunzel's sign). The presence of a cremasteric reflex almost always rules out testicular torsion.
3. Relief of pain by elevation of the affected testis (Prehn's sign) suggests epididymitis. A negative Prehn's sign (elevation of the testis does not relieve the pain) suggests testicular torsion.

### G. Diagnostic Imaging Tests
1. Diagnostic testing should not delay surgical exploration in acute torsion. If the diagnosis is unclear, diagnostic tests may be useful.
2. Color Doppler ultrasound has emerged as the most valuable diagnostic study, with nearly 100% sensitivity and specificity.
3. Surgical exploration remains the best diagnostic tool.

### H. Management of Testicular Torsion
1. Immediate detorsion is imperative for all cases of testicular torsion. Testicular salvage rates decrease to 50% at 10 hours and to 10-20% at 24 hours.
2. Manual detorsion can be attempted as an urgent measure by rotating the testicle about its pedicle. Surgical orchiopexy, however, is still required.
3. If an infarcted testicle is noted during surgical exploration, it should be removed. If the testicle is viable, both testicles should be fixed in the scrotum with nonabsorbable sutures.

## III. Priapism
### A. Priapism is defined as a prolonged penile erection.
### B. Most cases of priapism in adults are idiopathic. However, priapism often occurs secondary to vasoactive injectable drugs used to treat impotence. In children the most common causes are sickle cell anemia, hematologic neoplasms (leukemia), and trauma.

### C. Evaluation of Priapism
1. Patients usually complain of a persistent, painful erection. They may have fever and voiding difficulties.
2. Physical examination should include a neurologic evaluation and perineal inspection for neoplasms. Examination of the penis usually reveals a flaccid glans despite rigid corpora cavernosa.
3. Hematologic studies should be performed to rule out sickle cell anemia and leukemia.

### D. Treatment of Priapism
1. Early treatment of priapism reduces the risk of fibrosis of the corpora cavernosa and subsequent long-term impotence, which may occur in up to 50% of patients.
2. Discomfort can be reduced with parenteral narcotic analgesics and sedation.
3. Detumescence may be achieved using cold compresses, ice packs, warm- or cold-water enemas, and prostate massage.
4. If these treatments are unsuccessful, the static blood may be aspirated from the corpora using a large bore needle. Followed by irrigation of the corpora with saline containing a vasoconstricting agent (phenylephrine, epinephrine, or metaraminol).
5. If this process fails to achieve detumescence, a shunt may be created between the affected corpora cavernosa and unaffected corpus spongiosum with a Tru-Cut biopsy needle.

6. When priapism is secondary to sickle cell anemia, therapy also includes hydration, oxygen, and blood transfusion.

# Vascular and Orthopedic Surgery

Ian L. Gordon, M.D., Ph.D.
Harry Skinner, M.D.

## Peripheral Arterial Disease

Peripheral arterial disease is characterized by intermittent claudication, consisting of exercise-induced lower extremity pain that is relieved by rest. Claudication occurs when the blood supply is inadequate to meet the demand of lower limb muscles as a result of atherosclerotic arterial stenosis.

I. **Pathophysiology**
   A. The incidence of claudication rises sharply between ages 50 and 75 years, particularly in persons with coronary artery disease.
   B. This condition affects at least 10% of persons over 70 years of age and 2% of those 37-69 years of age.
   C. **Risk factors**
      1. Cigarette smoking is the most important risk factor for PAD. 70-90% of patients with arterial insufficiency are smokers. Risk remains increased for up to 5 years after smoking cessation.
      2. Other risk factors include hyperlipidemia, diabetes mellitus, and hypertension.
   D. After five-years, 4% of patients with claudication lose a limb and 16% have worsening claudication or limb-threatening ischemia.
   E. The five-year mortality rate for patients with claudication is 29%; 60% of deaths result from coronary artery disease, 15% from cerebrovascular disease, and the remainder result from nonatherosclerotic causes.

II. **Clinical Evaluation of Claudication**
   A. Evaluation consists of determining the location, extent, and severity of disease and the degree of functional impairment.
   B. **Claudication**
      1. The key clinical features of claudication are reproducibility of muscular pain in the thigh or calf after a given level of activity, and cessation of pain after a period of rest.
      2. Patients should be asked about the intensity of claudication, its location, and the distance they have to walk before it begins.
      3. **Aortoiliac disease** is manifest by discomfort in buttock and/or thigh and may result in impotence and reduced femoral pulses. **Leriche's syndrome** occurs when impotence is associated with bilateral hip or thigh claudication.
      4. **Iliofemoral occlusive disease** is characterized by thigh and calf claudication. Pulses are diminished from the groin to the foot.
      5. **Femoropopliteal disease** usually causes calf pain. Patients have normal groin pulses but diminished pulses distally.
      6. **Tibial vessel occlusive disease** may lead to foot claudication, rest pain, non-healing wounds, and gangrene.
         a. **Rest pain** consists of severe pain in the distal portion of foot due to ischemic neuritis.

## Peripheral Arterial Disease

    b. The pain is deep and unremitting, and it is exacerbated by elevation and relieved by dangling the affected foot over the side of the bed.

### III. Physical Examination
   A. **Evaluation of the Peripheral Pulses** should include the femoral, popliteal, posterior tibial, and dorsalis pedis arteries. The quality of the pulse and any pulse asymmetries between the limbs should be noted.
   B. Other signs of chronic arterial insufficiency include brittle nails, scaling skin, hair loss on the foot and lower leg, cold feet, cyanosis, and muscle atrophy. Careful inspection of the foot for skin breakdown or ulceration is important.
   C. Bruits may be auscultated distal to the arterial obstruction.
   D. Abdominal examination for a "pulsatile mass" is performed because of the strong association between abdominal aortic aneurysm and peripheral arterial disease.

### IV. Differential Diagnosis
   A. **Neurogenic Claudication (spinal stenosis)**
   1. Neurogenic claudication is the clinical syndrome most difficult to distinguish from claudication. Neurogenic claudication is caused by osteophytic narrowing of the neural canal around the spinal nerves.
   2. This syndrome causes radicular leg pain that begins with a change of posture and is relieved by assuming the recumbent position. The leg pain is often accompanied by burning, tingling, and numbness.
   3. The pain of neurogenic claudication persists even after the patient has stopped walking or occurs with mere standing or after prolonged sitting. With neurogenic claudication, the distance walked until the onset of pain varies.
   B. **Nocturnal muscle cramps** occur in older persons, but the cramps are not related to exercise.
   C. **Chronic compartment syndrome** may occur in young athletes characterized by tightness and pain in the calf after vigorous exercise. The pain does not quickly subside with rest.
   D. **Osteoarthritis of the hip** may mimic thigh and buttock claudication. However, osteoarthritic pain occurs with variable amounts of exercise,, and the pain changes in severity from day to day.

### V. Laboratory Testing of Arterial Disease
   A. **Ankle-brachial Index (ABI)**
   1. The ankle-brachial index (ABI) is the ratio of ankle systolic blood pressure to arm systolic blood pressure. It is highly sensitive and specific for peripheral arterial disease in nondiabetic patients.
      a. 0.75 is considered normal
      b. 0.40-0.75 suggests arterial obstruction with claudication
      c. <0.40 suggests significant arterial obstruction with critical ischemia (ie, non-healing wounds or rest pain).
   2. Patients occasionally have normal ABIs at rest, but their symptoms strongly suggest claudication. In these patients, ABIs should be obtained before and after exercise. Exercise may unmask obstruction.
   3. ABI and segmental blood pressure measurements are not accurate in patients with calcified vessels (especially diabetics) because ankle blood pressure readings tend to be falsely elevated.
   B. **Color Doppler imaging** is a good diagnostic alternative for patients at high risk for calcification of vessels.

- **C. Arteriography** is indicated following evaluation of ABIs if a patient with claudication is to undergo surgical or endovascular treatment.
- **D. Magnetic resonance angiography** has superior sensitivity over conventional angiography in detecting disease in distal runoff vessels.

## VI. Management of Peripheral Arterial Disease

- **A. Risk Factor Modification**
    1. **Cigarette smoking** is the most important modifiable risk factor. Claudication patients who abstain from tobacco usually do not progress to limb loss, whereas 11.3% of the patients who continue smoking require amputation.
    2. **Meticulous care of skin** of the lower limbs helps avoid ulcer formation and skin infection.
    3. **Obese patients** should be advised to lose weight through exercise and diet.
    4. **Hypertension** should be vigorously treated. Beta-blockers do not usually worsen claudication.
    5. **Hyperlipidemia.** Regression of femoral atherosclerosis is possible with lipid-lowering therapy. The goal should be to lower the low-density lipoprotein cholesterol level to below 100 mg/dL.
    6. **Diabetes** should be aggressively controlled in order to prevent further complications of microvascular disease.
- **B. Coronary and carotid artery disease assessment** is essential because coronary disease accounts for 60% of deaths.
- **C. Hormone replacement therapy** after menopause may slow the progression of atherosclerosis.
- **D. Progressive Exercise Training**
    1. Patients who have intermittent claudication but no rest pain or ischemic ulceration should begin a walking program. They can usually increase their walking distance several times above baseline and can usually reduce the pain of claudication.
    2. Patients should walk to or through the onset of claudication, rest until the pain resolves, and then resume exercise; 30 minutes every day.
- **E. Pharmacologic Management**
    1. **Pentoxifylline (Trental)**
        a. The effect of pentoxifylline is only modest. Patients who take it may have a 20% increase in walking distance; however, exercise alone may increase walking distance up to 25%. This drug is useful only in patients who cannot benefit from exercise.
        b. Pentoxifylline is given in a dose of 400 mg tid. Gastrointestinal side effects may occur.
    2. **Aspirin** has no effect on claudication, but because of the high incidence of cerebrovascular and cardiovascular disease, aspirin, 160-325 mg per day, should be given.
- **F. Operative and Endovascular Procedures**
    1. Most patients with claudication respond to conservative therapy. Surgery is reserved for patients with rest pain or tissue loss. Patients who have intermittent calf claudication alone are not surgical candidates unless the claudication severely limits their lifestyle or occupational functioning.
    2. Patients with rest pain, tissue loss as a result of gangrene, or non-healing ulcers, with an ABI in the range of 0.3, are surgical candidates.
    3. Percutaneous transluminal angioplasty has a greater than 90%

success rate in the treatment of short-segment aortoiliac occlusive disease, and these results may be improved with the placement of an intra-arterial stent. However, five-year patency rates are only 40-60%.
    4. Surgical bypass therapy is an effective treatment for claudication; however, it is associated with 5-10% morbidity and mortality rates. Aortobifemoral grafting has a 90% 5-year patency rate. Aortoiliac, femoral-femoral crossover, and reversed and in-situ saphenous vein bypass grafting from the common femoral to the popliteal artery have 60-70% 5-year patency rates. A synthetic polytetrafluoroethylene graft (PTFE) is indicated for above knee femoral-popliteal bypass, and it has a 50% 5-year patency rate.
  G. **Axillofemoral Bypass.** This procedure is useful for high risk, elderly patients who are unable to tolerate an aortic procedure.
VII. **Management of the Acutely Threatened Limb**
  A. An acutely occluded artery can result in limb loss within hours. The patient will complain of sudden onset of severe unrelenting rest pain. Atrial fibrillation often may cause an acute embolic arterial occlusion.
  B. These patients require emergency surgical evaluation and immediate heparinization.

**References:** See page 106.

# Deep Venous Thrombosis

I. **Pathophysiology**
  A. Fifty percent of venous thrombi of the lower extremity will embolize to the lung if not treated. The source of symptomatic pulmonary emboli is usually thrombosis in the larger veins above the knee rather than thrombosis in the veins of the calf.
  B. Deep venous thrombosis can be found in at least 80% of patients with a pulmonary emboli.
II. **Risk Factors for Deep Venous Thrombosis**
  A. **Venous Stasis** risk factors include prolonged immobilization, stroke, myocardial infarction, heart failure, obesity, varicose veins, anesthesia, age >65 years old.
  B. **Endothelial Injury** risk factors include surgery, trauma, central venous access catheters, pacemaker wires, previous thromboembolic event (especially if precipitating factors are not eliminated).
  C. **Hypercoagulable State** risk factors include malignant disease, high estrogen level (pregnancy, oral contraceptives).
  D. **Hematologic Disorders.** Polycythemia, leukocytosis, thrombocytosis, antithrombin III deficiency, protein C deficiency, protein S deficiency, antiphospholipid syndrome, inflammatory bowel disease.
III. **Signs and Symptoms of Deep Venous Thrombosis**
  A. Signs and symptoms of DVT are absent in about 50%, and they range from subtle to obvious.
  B. The disorder may be asymptomatic, or the patient may complain of pain, swelling, "heaviness," aching, or the sudden appearance of varicose veins. Risk factors may be absent.
  C. DVT may manifest as a unilaterally edematous limb with a erythrocyanotic appearance, dilated superficial veins, elevated skin temperature, tenderness in the thigh or calf. Absence of clinical signs does not preclude

# Deep Venous Thrombosis

the diagnosis.
- **D.** A swollen, tender leg with a palpable venous "cord" in the popliteal fossa strongly suggests popliteal DVT. Marked discrepancy in limb circumference supports the diagnosis of DVT, but most patients do not have measurable swelling.
- **E.** The clinical diagnosis of DVT is correct only 50% of the time; therefore, diagnostic testing is mandatory when DVT is suspected.

## IV. Diagnostic Testing
- **A. Impedance Plethysmography** depends on the detection of impaired venous emptying of the leg. It has a high false negative rate, and over 30% of cases may be missed. Plethysmography is used in conjunction with duplex scanning.
- **B. Duplex Scanning**
    1. When Doppler measurement of blood flow is added to ultrasound imaging, the combination is referred to as a duplex scan.
    2. **Doppler Studies:** Uses Doppler shifts to detect blood flow in the veins.
    3. **Ultrasound Imaging.** Two-dimensional ultrasonography produces an image of the deep veins.
- **C.** When results of impedance plethysmography and duplex scanning are positive, these techniques are adequately specific to diagnose DVT. Results that do not support the clinical impression should be investigated with venography.
- **D. Contrast Venography**
    1. When impedance plethysmography and ultrasound techniques fail to demonstrate a thrombus, venography is the diagnostic "gold standard" for patients at high clinical risk. The test is negative if contrast medium is seen throughout the deep venous system.
    2. Venography can cause iatrogenic venous thrombosis in 4%, and allergic contrast reactions occur in 3% of patients.
- **E. MRI** may have an accuracy comparable to that of contrast venography, and it may soon replace contrast venography as the "gold standard" of venous imaging.

## V. Treatment of Deep Vein Thrombosis
- **A. Heparin Anticoagulation**
    1. Anticoagulant therapy should be initiated as soon as venous thrombosis is clinically recognized as likely, while awaiting the completion of a diagnostic workup.
    2. **Initial Bolus.** 10,000 U of heparin by intravenous push
    3. **Initial Maintenance Drip**
        a. Mix 20,000 U of heparin in 500 cc of D5W or normal saline (40 U/cc)
        b. Start drip beginning at 32 cc/hr (1,280 U/hr)
    4. Check aPTT 6 hr after giving initial bolus.
    5. **Therapeutic Range.** Activated PTT 1.5-2.0 times control.
    6. The amount of heparin needed for effective anticoagulation is higher than was once used; a 5,000-U bolus and a drip of 1,000 U/hr usually does not produce a therapeutic aPTT within the first 48 hours.

## Maintenance Dose Adjustment

| aPTT | Hold drip | Adjust drip | Check aPTT |
| --- | --- | --- | --- |
| <50 sec | 0 min | Increase 3 cc/hr | 6 hr later |
| 50-59 sec | 0 min | Increase 3 cc/hr | 6 hr later |
| 60-85 sec | 0 min | No change | Next morning |
| 86-95 sec | 0 min | Decrease 2 cc/hr | Next morning |
| 96-120 sec | 30 min | Decrease 2 cc/hr | 6 hr later |
| >120 sec | 60 min | Decrease 4 cc/hr | 6 hr later |

1. Heparin must be continued until the anticoagulant effects of warfarin have become established (usually 3 to 5 days after initiation).
2. Monitor platelet count during heparin therapy; thrombocytopenia develops in up to 5%. Heparin rarely induces hyperkalemia, which resolves spontaneously upon discontinuation. Ambulation can begin once the activated PTT is in the therapeutic range.

### A. Warfarin (Coumadin)
1. Oral anticoagulants should be started only after effective anticoagulation with heparin has been established because they increase coagulability and thrombogenesis during the first few days of administration. There is a high incidence of embolization when oral warfarin is started without adequate prior heparinization.
2. **Warfarin**, initial dose 10 mg PO qd; subsequent doses should be based on a daily PT values and its rate of change.
3. After heparin therapy has overlapped with warfarin therapy for 3-5 days and the international normalized ratio is 2.0-3.0 (INR), heparin can be safely discontinued. Outpatients receiving oral anticoagulants should have their INR checked weekly.
4. **Length of Warfarin Therapy.** Oral anticoagulation should be maintained for 3 months after a first episode of DVT or pulmonary embolism. Indications to prolong therapy to 6-12 months include persistent risk factors, extensive or complicated thrombosis, or recurrent thrombotic episodes.

### B. Thrombolytic Therapy
1. Thrombolytics clear the thrombus more rapidly.
2. Thrombolytics are indicated only for severe venous outflow obstruction (phlegmasia cerulea dolens).
3. **Contraindications to Thrombolytics**
   a. **Absolute Contraindications.** Active bleeding, recent stroke, central nervous system tumor.
   b. **Relative Contraindications.** Surgical procedure within preceding 10 days; recent gastrointestinal bleeding; uncontrolled hypertension; recent trauma, pregnancy, endocarditis, renal or hepatic failure, left-sided heart thrombus.
4. The thrombus should usually be demonstrated by venography before thrombolytics are used.

5. **Streptokinase.** Duration required for complete clot lysis is substantially longer with streptokinase than with tissue plasminogen activator (tPA); much less expensive than tPA. **Dosage:** bolus of 250,000 U IV followed by 100,000 U/hr
6. **Tissue Plasminogen Activator.** tPA is "clot-selective", and may promote clot lysis more rapidly than other agents. **Dosage:** 100 mg over a 2-3 hour period.

C. **Vena Caval Interruption Methods**
1. Pulmonary embolism can be prevented by percutaneous filter interruption of the inferior vena cava. Filters have a patency rate of 95% and are effective in preventing 95% of emboli.
2. **Indications for Vena Cava Filter.** Pulmonary embolism despite adequate anticoagulation, contraindications to anticoagulants, prevention of recurrent pulmonary embolism in high-risk patients.

**References:** See page 106.

# Orthopedic Fractures and Dislocations

I. **Clinical Evaluation of the Injured Limb**
A. **Physical Examination of the Injured Limb.** 1) Inspection--look, 2) Palpation -- feel, and 3) Movement -- move. Specifically examine the bone for instability and examine the soft tissue for associated injury. Evaluate and document neurologic and vascular status.
B. **Clinical Features of Fractures**
1. **Pain and Tenderness.** All fractures cause pain in the neurologically intact limb.
2. **Loss of Function.** Pain and loss of structural integrity of the limb causes loss of function.
3. **Deformity.** Change in length, angulation, rotation and displacement.
4. **Attitude.** The position of the fractured limb is sometimes diagnostic. For example the patient with a fractured clavicle usually supports the limb and rotates his head to the affected side.
5. **Abnormal Mobility and Crepitus:** Eliciting these signs may be painful and dangerous, and they should not be sought deliberately.
C. **Clinical Features of Dislocations**
1. A dislocation occurs when the articular surfaces of a joint are no longer in contact. Subluxation (partial dislocation) is a less severe condition that occurs when the orientation of the surfaces is altered but they remain in contact.
2. **Pain and Tenderness.** Severe pain may be completely relieved when the joint is relocated.
3. **Loss of Motion.** Both active and passive motion are limited in all dislocations.
4. **Loss of Normal Joint Contour.** In the anteriorly dislocated shoulder, the deltoid is flattened and the greater tuberosity of the humerus is no longer lateral to the acromion.
5. **Attitude.** The patient carefully holds the anteriorly dislocated shoulder in abduction and external rotation.
6. **Neurologic Injury.** The incidence of neurologic injuries is much higher with dislocations than with fractures. Shoulder dislocations are often associated with axillary nerve injury. Posterior dislocations of the

hip can result in sciatic nerve contusion. Careful examination for neurologic status is indicated before any intervention. If a neurologic injury is caused by the reduction maneuver, immediate open exploration is indicated.

## II. Clinical Description of Fractures

### A. Anatomic Location
1. **Metaphyseal** -- Fracture through metaphysis
2. **Diaphyseal** -- Fracture through diaphysis (proximal, middle or distal third of the shaft)
3. **Epiphyseal** -- Fracture through epiphysis or physis
4. **Salter Classification of Fractures (children only):**
   **Type I:** Fracture through physis, between the epiphysis and metaphysis
   **Type II:** Fracture through physis, involving the metaphysis
   **Type III:** Fracture through physis, involving the epiphysis
   **Type IV:** Fracture through physis, involving the metaphysis and epiphysis
   **Type V:** Crush injury to physis, between the epiphysis and metaphysis

### B. Bony Deformity.
Describe any change in bone length, angulation, rotation, and displacement.

### C. Direction of the fracture line.
Describe the radiographic direction of the fracture.
1. **Transverse** -- Perpendicular to the long axis of the bone
2. **Oblique** -- Fracture is at an angle to the bone
3. **Spiral** -- Secondary to torsional stress

### D. Comminution.
Fracture with more than two fragments.

### E. Open vs Closed.
In an open fracture the bone protrudes through the skin.

### F. Buckle Fracture.
One cortex is broken while the other remains intact.

## III. Radiologic Evaluation of Fractures

### A.
A minimum of two views at right angles to each other should be obtained. Visualize the joint above and below the injury and check for soft tissue swelling.

### B.
Views of the uninjured extremity are often useful for comparison in children.

## IV. Management of Fractures

### A. Fracture Reduction
1. The fracture must be restored to a normal anatomical position.
2. Muscle spasm should be relieved with traction, analgesics, muscle relaxants.
3. Bones must be in apposition, properly aligned in linear and rotary directions, and set to proper length.

### B. Indications for Operative Treatment
1. **Failure of closed methods** to reduce the fracture.
2. **Multiple Injuries.** Multiple fractures should be fixed internally.
3. **Early Mobilization.** Associated medical problems and high cost can be avoided by early mobilization.
4. **Fractured and Displaced Articular Surfaces.** Operative treatment minimizes the risk of late degenerative changes.

### C. Upper Extremity Fractures and Dislocations
1. **Clavicle Fractures.** Cannot be casted. Subclavian artery and brachial

plexus injury may occur. Splint with figure-of-eight bandage, or if figure of eight causes posterior angulation, use triangular sling.
2. **Humerus Fractures.** X-ray the entire bone, and check for radial nerve injury (wrist drop). Treat with collar-and-cuff sling; immobilize the joints above and below fracture.
3. **Anterior Shoulder Dislocation.** The humeral head has been forced anterior to glenoid. Usually caused by extension force applied to abducted arm. Patient presents with arm in slight abduction and cannot bring elbow to side; there is a slightly depressed deltoid prominence, and arm motion causes pain. Axillary nerve injury may occur, causing a sensory deficit over the deltoid. Reduce with gentle traction.
4. **Posterior Shoulder Dislocation.** The humeral head has been forced posterior to the glenoid. May be secondary to seizures or electrocution. Reduce with gentle traction.
5. **Colles Fracture.** Distal radius is angulated dorsally; associated fracture of the ulnar styloid. Treatment consists of reduction, casting, and elevation of the extremity until swelling subsides; check alignment with a postreduction x-ray; rule out median nerve injury by examination.
6. **Smith Fracture.** Volar angulation of the fractured radius (reverse Colles). This fracture should be reduced and cast in the same manner as a Colles fracture in slight flexion. Frequently surgical fixation is necessary because the fracture is unstable.

D. **Lower Extremity Fractures and Dislocations**
1. **Femoral Neck Fractures.** Osteoporotic bone predisposes to this intracapsular fracture. Internal fixation or endoprostheses (artificial hip) are required.
2. **Intertrochanteric Fractures.** Usually occurs in elderly after a fall out of bed. The fracture is located on the outside of the joint capsule. Internal fixation is required.
3. **Femoral Shaft Fracture.** May occasionally cause an arterial injury. Early intramedullary nailing is recommended in adults.

E. **Knee Injuries**
1. **Knee Ligament Testing**
    a. **Varus/Valgus Stress of the Tibia on the Femur.** Examiner stabilizes the femur, and pressure is exerted outward or inward at the ankle; a tear of the collateral ligament is indicated by excess mobility.
    b. **Anterior Drawer Test.** Pull tibia anteriorly with the knee flexed 90° (tests for tear of anterior cruciate).
    c. **Posterior Drawer Test.** Push tibia posteriorly with the knee flexed 90° (tests for tear of posterior cruciate).
2. The most common ligamentous injuries are tearing of the medial collateral ligament, by a blow from the lateral side of the knee, and tear of the anterior cruciate ligament injury by twisting on a planted foot. Brace immobilization is usually sufficient.
3. Dislocation of the knee often results in multiple ligament injury. Rule out popliteal artery trauma. Immobilization of the knee, followed by ligament reconstruction should be completed.

**References**
References may be obtained via the internet at www.CCSPublishing.com.

# Index

Abdominal trauma 28
Abdominal wall layers 54
ABI 98
Acute abdomen 49
Acute Abdomen management 51
Acute Blood Loss 13
Admitting orders 7
Albumin 13
American Surgical Association 8
Amikacin 18
Amikin 18
Amoxicillin 62
Ampicillin/Sulbactam 18
Amylase 77
Ancef 10
Anectine 41, 43
Angiodysplasia 66
Angiography 66
Ankle-brachial Index 98
Anorectal Disorders 68
Anterior Drawer Test 105
Anterior Nasal Pack 46
Antibiotic preparation for colonic surgery 7
Antrectomy 64
Aortic Transection 37
Aortoiliac disease 97
Appendectomy 53
Appendicitis 52
Arterial Line Placement 24
ASA 8
Aspirin 99
Astler-Coller Modification 73
Ativan 43
Atracurium 43
Axillofemoral Bypass 100
Axid Pulvules 63
Azactam 18
Aztreonam 18
B12 20
Bassini Repair 55
Beck's Triad 35
Biaxin 62
Billroth I 64
Billroth II 64
Bismuth 62
Bleeding Scan 66
Blood Component Therapy 12
Blood Replacement 27
Blunt Abdominal Trauma 29
Breast biopsy 87
Breast Cancer 85
Breast Mass 85
Breast Masses 85
Brief operative note 8
Burns 38
Calculi 91
Caput medusae 50
Carafate 63
Carcinoembryonic antigen 72
Cardiac Contusions 37
Cardiac Tamponade 35
Cefazolin 10
Cefizox 18
Cefotan 18
Cefotaxime 18

Cefotetan 18
Cefoxitin 10, 18, 79
Ceftazidime 18
Ceftizoxime 18
Central line 12
Central venous catheter 21
Central Venous Catheters 12
Charcot's sign 5
Charcot's triad 80
Chest Tube 12, 33
Chest Tube Insertion 33
Chief Compliant 5
Cholecystectomy 81
Cholecystitis 80
Cholelithiasis 80
Cimetidine 59, 63, 79
Claforan 18
Clarithromycin 62
Claudication 97
Clindamycin 18
Colles Fracture 105
Colloid 13
Colon Polyps 67
Colonoscopy 66
Colorectal Cancer 71
CoLyte 65
Compazine 10
Condylomata acuminata 70
Cooper's Ligament 54
Cooper's Ligament Repair 55
Coumadin 102
Courvoisier's sign 50
Cranial Nerve Examination 6
Cricothyrotomy 24
Crystalloids 12
Cullen's sign 50
Cutaneous hyperesthesia 52
CVAT 6
Cyst Aspiration 86
Deep tendon reflexes 6
Deep venous thrombosis 100
Demerol 81
Diagnostic Peritoneal Lavage 30
Diazepam 43
Diphenoxylate 19
Diprivan 43
Direct Inguinal Hernia 54
Discharge summary 11
Dislocations 103
Diverticulosis 66
Dobutamine 17
Dopamine 17
Doppler imaging 98
Doppler Studies 101
Dukes' Classification 73
Duodenal Ulcer Disease 63
Duplex Scanning 101
Electrolytes 12
Endotracheal tube 12, 41
Enteral feeding 19
Epigastric Hernia 55
Epinephrine 17
Epistaxis 44
Erythromycin 7

Esophageal Injuries 37
External Hemorrhoids 69
External Inguinal Ring 54
External oblique 54
Extremity Fractures 37
Famotidine 59, 63
Femoral Canal 54
Femoral Hernia 54
Femoral Hernia Repair 55
Femoral Neck Fractures 105
Femoral Shaft Fracture 105
Fentanyl 41
Fever 14
Fine-Needle Aspiration 86
Fine-Needle Aspiration Cytology 86
First Degree Burns 39
Fistula-in-Ano 71
Fistulectomy 71
Fistulotomy 71
Flagyl 18, 62, 81
Flail Chest 34
Floxin 18
Fluids 13
Flutamide 90
Fortaz 18
Fractures 103
Fresh Frozen Plasma 13
Gastric Ulcer 64
Gastroduodenostomy 64
Gastrojejunostomy 63, 64
Gentamicin 18, 81
Glasgow Coma Scale 31
GoLYTELY 7
Goodsall's rule 71
Gun Shot Wounds 29
Halsted Repair 55
Head Trauma 31
  Emergency Management 31
  Open Head Injury 32
Helicobacter pylori 61
Hematemesis 58
Hematochezia 49, 64
Hemorrhoids 67, 68
Hemothorax 35
Heparin 101
Hernia 54
Hernia classification 54
Hernia repair techniques 55
Hesselbach's Triangle 54
History of Present Illness 5
Humerus Fractures 105
Iliopsoas sign 50
Impedance Plethysmography 101
Impotence 97
Incarcerated hernia 54, 56
Incisional Hernia 55
Indirect Hernia 56
Indirect Inguinal Hernia 54
Inflammatory Bowel Disease 67
Inguinal anatomy 54
Inguinal Ligament 54
Internal Hemorrhoids 68

Internal Jugular Vein Cannulation 21
Internal oblique 54
Internal Ring 54
Intertrochanteric Fractures 105
Intestinal obstruction 75
Intravenous Pyelogram 91
Intubation 41, 42
Ischemic Colitis 67
Knee Injuries 105
Lacunar Ligament 54
Lansoprazole 63
Laparoscopic Cholecystectomy 82
Leriche's syndrome 97
Leuprolide 90
Linton-Nachlas tube 60
Lipase 78
Lomotil 19
Lorazepam 43
Lower Gastrointestinal Bleeding 64
Mallory-Weiss Syndrome 59
McBurney's point 50, 52
McVay Repair 55
Mefoxin 18, 79
Melena 49, 64
Mesenteric ischemia 74
Metoclopramide 7
Metronidazole 18, 62, 63, 81
Metronidazole 7
Mezlocillin 18
Midazolam 41-43
Morphine 43
Murphy's sign 80
Murphy's Sign 14
Nasal Pack 46
Nasogastric Tubes 12
Nasotracheal Intubation 42
Neo-Synephrine 42
Neomycin 7
Nizatidine 63
Norcuron 43
Norepinephrine 17
Obstipation 49
Obturator Hernia 55
Obturator sign 50
Octreotide 60, 79
Ofloxacin 18
Omeprazole 62, 63
Operative report 9
Oral antibiotic prep 7
Orchiectomy 90
Osmolytic 19
Packed Red Blood Cells 13
Pancreatitis 76
Pancuronium 43
Pantaloon Hernia 54
Parenteral Nutrition 19
Past Medical History 5
Pavulon 43
Pelvic Fracture 37
Penetrating Abdominal Trauma 29
Pentoxifylline 99
Pepcid 59, 63
Peptic ulcer disease 61
PeptoBismol 62
Perianal Abscess 69
Pericardiocentesis 36
Perineal Hernia 55
Peripheral Arterial Disease 97
Peripheral parenteral nutrition 20
Peritoneal Hernia Repair 55
Peritoneal Lavage 30
PERRLA 5
Petit's Hernia 55
Phenylephrine 17, 42
Piperacillin 18
Piperacillin/tazobactam 18
Piperacillin/tazobactam 81
Pitressin 60
Platelets 13
Pneumothorax 32
Polyethylene glycol solution 7
Post-Operative Note 9
Post-Operative Management 10
Post-Operative Orders 9
Posterior Drawer Test 105
Posterior Pack 47
Postoperative Fever Workup 14
Postural hypotension 58
Preoperative note 8
Preoperative orders 7
Preoperative preparation 6
Prevacid 63
Priapism 95
Prilosec 62, 63
Primary Survey 27
Problem-oriented progress note 10
Processus Vaginalis 54
Prochlorperazine 10
Propofol 43
Prostate Cancer 88
Prostate Specific Antigen 88
Prostate Specific Antigen Levels 88
PSA 88
Pseudocyst 79, 80
Pulmonary Artery Catheter Values 23
Pulmonary Artery Catheterization 22
Pulmonary Artery Catheters 12
Pulmonary Contusions 37
Pulmonology 41
Pulses 6
Pyloroplasty 63
Quinupristin/dalfopristin 18
Radiographic Evaluation 12
Ranitidine 59, 62, 63, 79
Ranitidine-bismuth-citrate 63
Ranson's Criteria 78
Rectus sheath 54
Red Blood Cell Transfusion 13
Reglan 20
Renal Calculi 91
Renal Colic 90
Rest Pain 97
Review of Systems 5
Richter's Hernia 54
Ringer's lactate 36
Rovsing's sign 50, 52
Salter Classification 104
Sandostatin 60, 61, 79
Scarpa's fascia 54
Sciatic Hernia 55
Secondary Survey 27
Sepsis 15, 17
Septic shock 15
Seton Procedure 71
Shoulder Dislocation 105
Sliding Hernia 54
Smith Fracture 105
Somatostatin 79
Sphincterotomy 69
Spigelian Hernia 55
Sponge Pack 47
Stab Wounds 29
Stigmata of Liver Disease 50
Strangulated Hernia 54
Streptokinase 103
Subclavian Vein Cannulation 22
Sublimaze 41
Succinylcholine 41, 43
Sucralfate 63
Surgical History 5
Surgical physical examination 5
Synercid 18
Tagamet 59, 63, 79
Tamponade 60
Targocid 18
Technetium Scan 66
Teicoplanin 18
Tension Pneumothorax 33
Testicular Torsion 94
Tetracycline 62
Ticarcillin 18
Ticarcillin/clavulanate 18
Ticarcillin/Clavulanic 81
Timentin 18, 81
Tissue Plasminogen Activator 103
TNM Classification 73
Tobramycin 18
Total parenteral nutrition 19
Tracheostomy 12
Tracrium 43
Transversalis fascia 54
Transversus abdominous 54
Trauma 27
Trental 99
Tritec 63
Ulcer 61
Umbilical Hernia 54
Unasyn 18
Upper Gastrointestinal Bleeding 58
Urea Breath Test 62
Urinary Retention 92, 93
Urine analysis 6
Urologic Emergencies 92
Vagotomy 63
Valium 43
Vancomycin 18
Variceal 61
Variceal bleeding 59
Vascular surgery 97
Vasopressin 60
Vecuronium 43
Venography 101
Venous Cutdown 23
Ventral Hernias 56
Versed 41-43

Vitamin B12 20
Warfarin 102
Whole gut lavage 7
Zantac 59, 62, 63, 79
Zosyn 18, 81

# Books from Current Clinical Strategies Publishing

## Available at Health Science Bookstores Worldwide

Practice Parameters in Medicine, Primary Care, and Family Practice, 1996 Edition

Handbook of Anesthesiology, 1997 Edition

Gynecology and Obstetrics, 1997 Edition

Manual of HIV/AIDS Therapy, 1997 Edition

Family Medicine, 1997 Edition

Surgery, 1997 Edition

Critical Care Medicine, 1997 Edition

Outpatient Medicine, 1997 Edition

Diagnostic History and Physical Exam in Medicine

Medicine, 1996 Edition

Handbook of Psychiatric Drugs, 1997 Edition

Psychiatry, 1997 Edition

Pediatrics, 1997 Edition

Physician's Drug Resource, 1997 Edition

Pediatric Drug Reference

## Windows, Macintosh, and Paperback

## http://www.CCSPublishing.com

## On-Line Journals from Current Clinical Strategies Publishing

Journal of Primary Care On-Line™
Journal of Medicine On-Line™
Journal of Pediatric Medicine On-Line™
Journal of Surgery On-Line™
Journal of Family Medicine On-Line™
Journal of Emergency Medicine On-Line™
Journal of Psychiatry On-Line™
Journal of AIDS and HIV™

http://www.CCSPublishing.com